MAKEUP.
FOR MEN

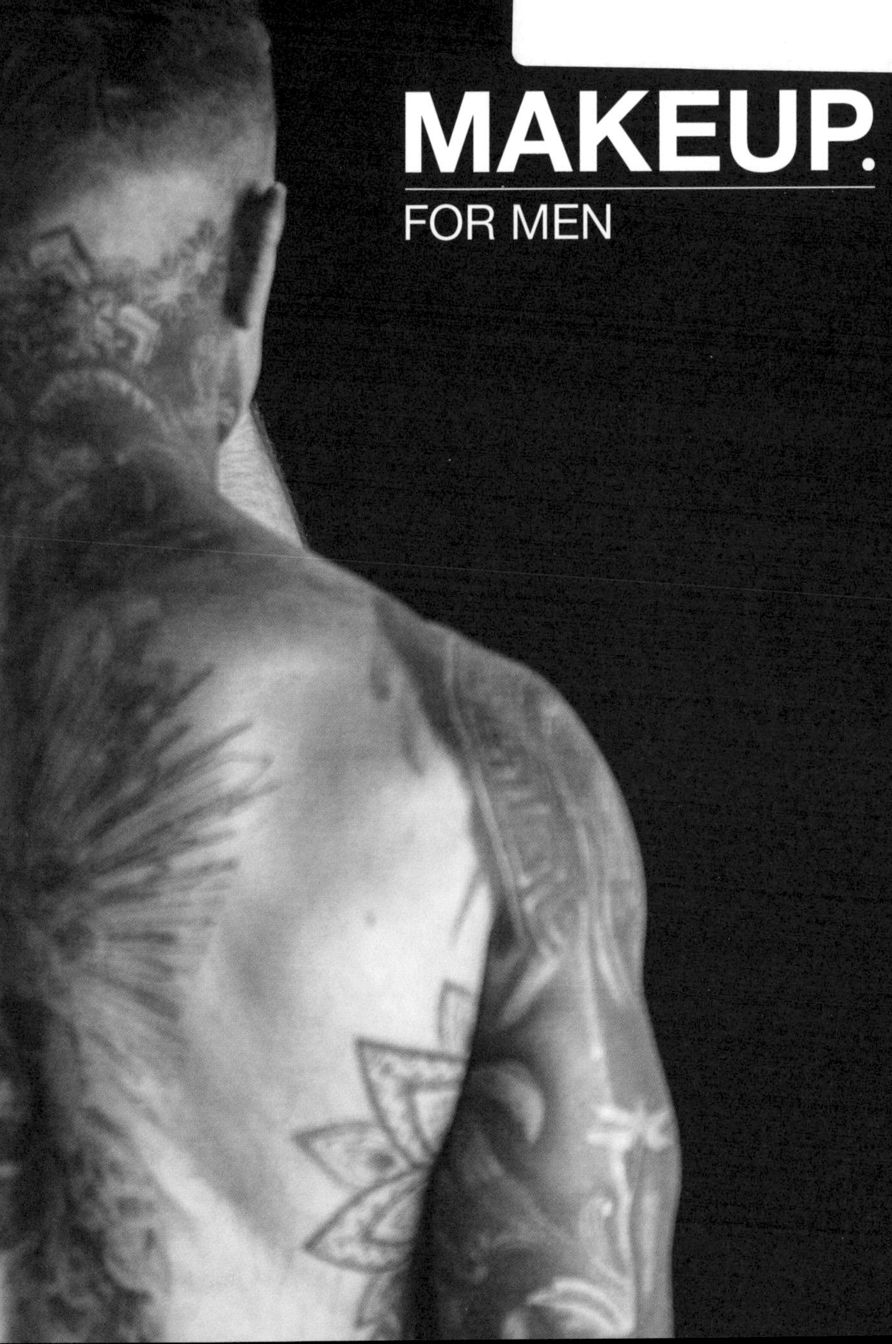

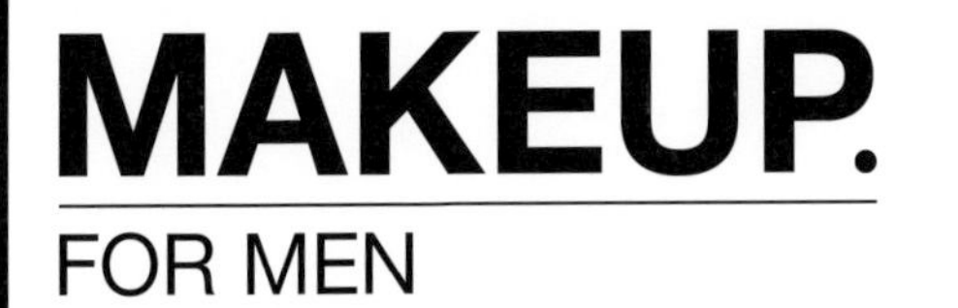

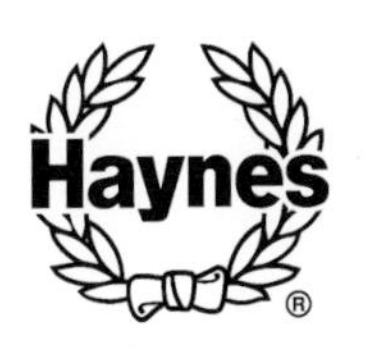

THE MANUAL FROM WAR PAINT.

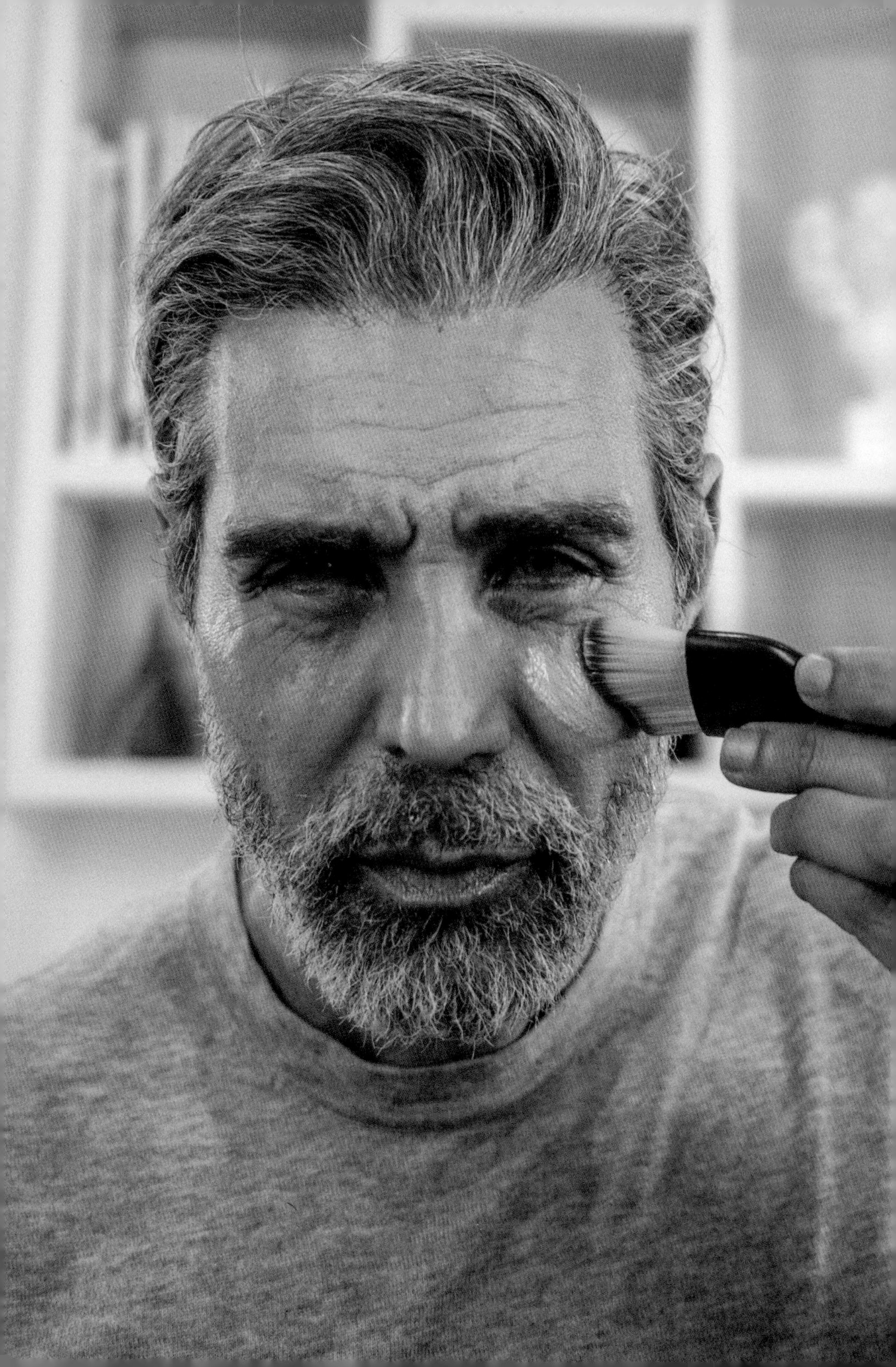

Contents

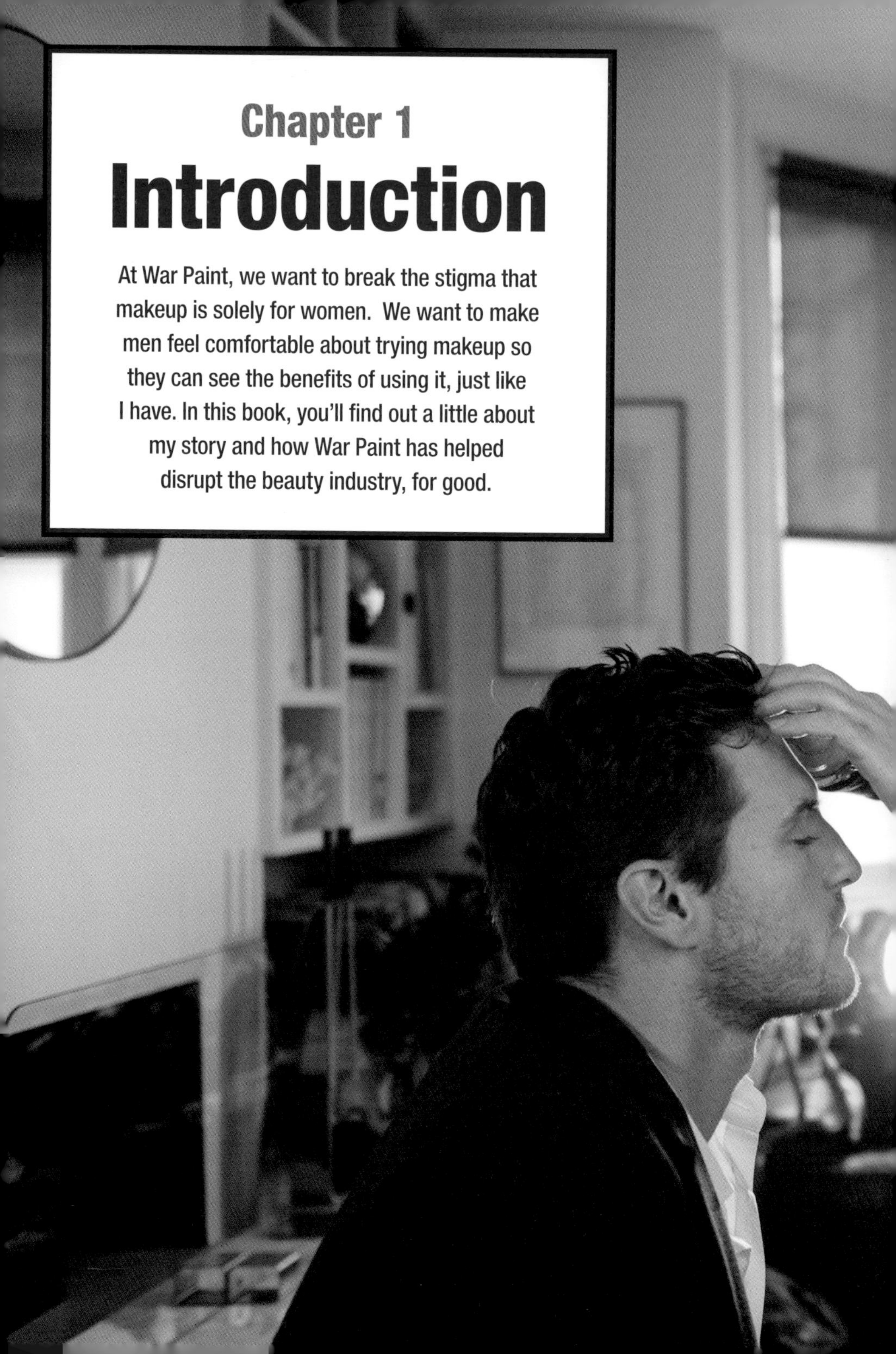

Chapter 1
Introduction

At War Paint, we want to break the stigma that makeup is solely for women. We want to make men feel comfortable about trying makeup so they can see the benefits of using it, just like I have. In this book, you'll find out a little about my story and how War Paint has helped disrupt the beauty industry, for good.

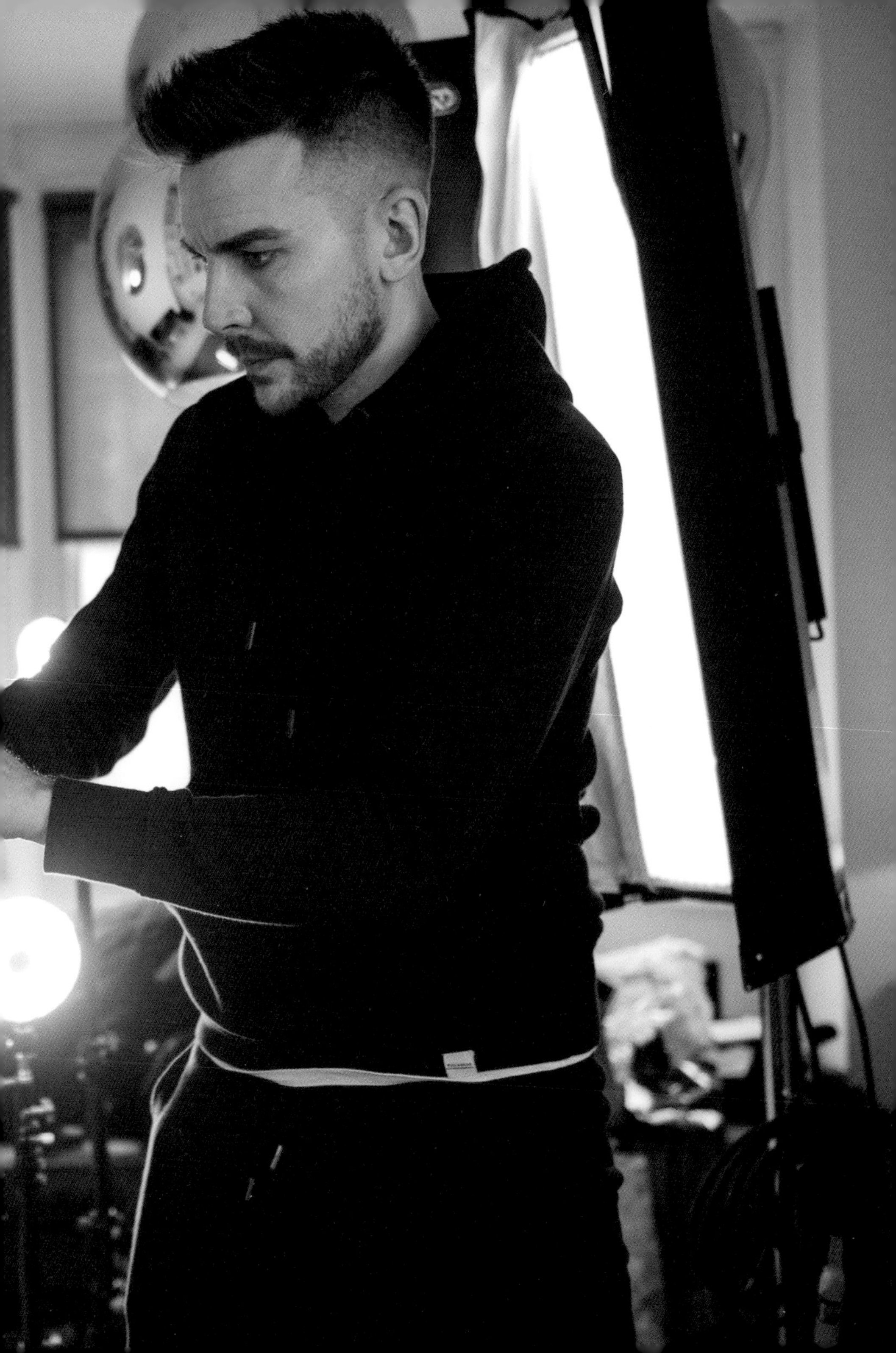

Meet Danny, founder of War Paint

My name is Danny Gray and I'm the founder of War Paint for Men. As the name suggests, it's a brand that's designed specifically for guys – simple products, applied in a simple way.

My aim is to change the whole thinking around men's makeup. I want it to become as normal and mundane as brushing your teeth.

The fact that you're reading this manual is a step in the right direction.

My story

War Paint is a really personal story for me. It started more than 20 years ago when I was bullied in middle school about my ears. I was 11 years old and those episodes of bullying in the school playground over a couple of weeks changed my life forever. I started developing a horrible feeling about going into school – and, worse, a horrible feeling about how I looked.

My anxiety about my appearance became so bad that my mum, Debbie, said there were times when she didn't know what to do to make things better.

I gradually started obsessing over the way I looked – so much so that I developed a form of body dysmorphia that still affects

↓ Danny, pictured aged 10, who was bullied at middle school because of his ears.

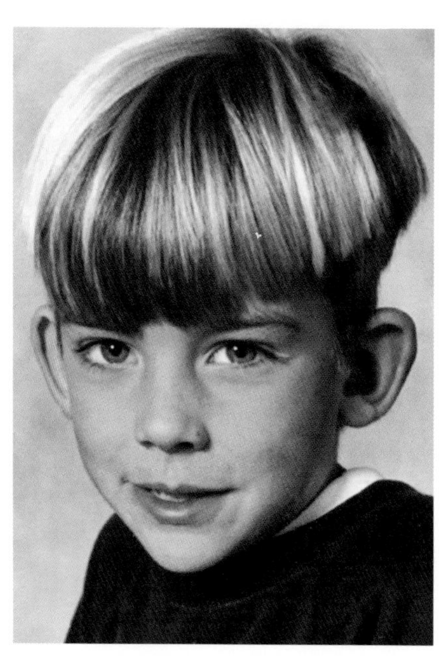

↓ Danny, aged 31, after his hair transplant procedure in 2017.

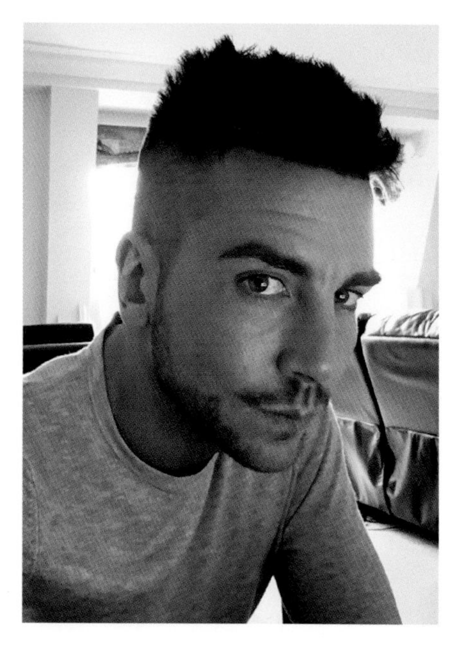

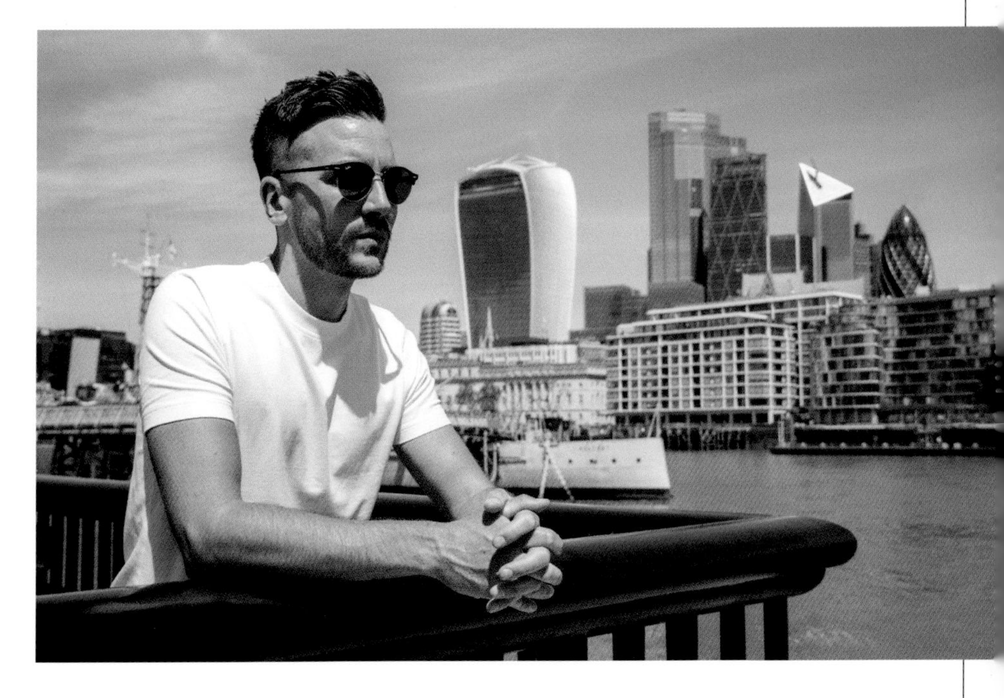

me today. Body dysmorphia is a mental health condition that causes people to spend a lot of time worrying about how they look. Gazing in the mirror can be confused with vanity, but the reality was that I was torturing myself with insecurities about my appearance. Mental health issues never leave you, you just learn to manage them. Let's be real here, I've had my ears pinned back twice, I've had a hair transplant and I use makeup – all tools that I've used to deal with my mental health and feel confident in myself again. I was told I didn't really need a hair transplant, but I had it done anyway and it transformed my life.

At 14 years old, like a lot of young guys, I started getting spots. With my body dysmorphia ramping up again, seeing my skin develop acne affected me pretty badly. I didn't want to go out. As my spots got worse, so too did my anxiety, so I turned to my sister for help. She handed me a concealer stick, showed me how to put it on, and it changed *everything*.

I couldn't believe the power of product and what it could do. That concealer gave me a glimmer of hope – it was a turning point. Using makeup helped build my confidence back up. Looking back, when I was getting acne, there were times when I wouldn't have been able to leave the house without makeup.

'I couldn't believe the power of product and what it could do. As somebody who suffers with body dysmorphia, that concealer gave me a glimmer of hope – it was a turning point.'

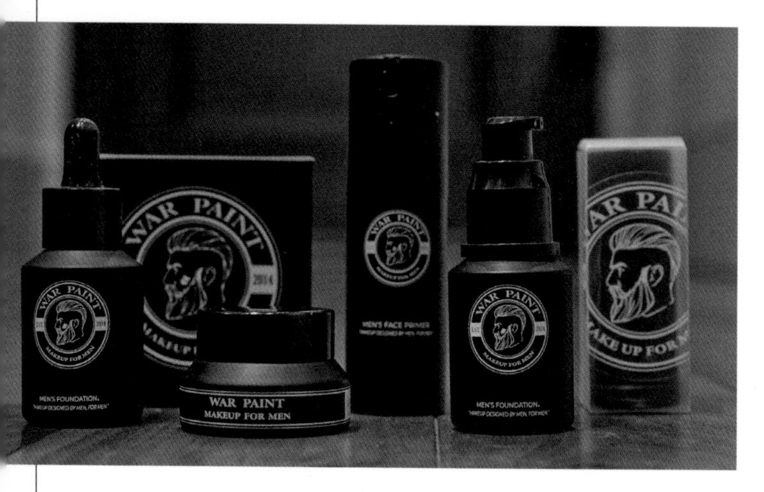

← Prototypes of the first War Paint makeup products that were used to test the market before launching. After a rebrand, War Paint launched in November 2018.

How War Paint started

War Paint wouldn't exist if I didn't have body dysmorphia. It's the reason why I started everything.

These days, my skin is acne-free but I still have a daily makeup routine – primer, foundation and sometimes bronzer because it makes me feel good. I've been wearing makeup for the last 20 years (I'm now in my mid-30s), but there were two things that I could never find as a man buying makeup: a brand that I could identify with, and somewhere I could go to try (and buy) products in confidence. That's why I started my own brand: War Paint for Men.

The idea first kicked off during a round of golf with my best mate. I had been going on and on about this gap in the market for men's makeup for more than a decade and he finally snapped when we were on the fifth hole and said to me, 'Danny, will you stop talking about it and just do it?' So I did. I lost that round of golf because my head was buzzing, but I went straight to my car and sat there for four hours calling people and trying to figure out how to get my idea off the ground.

I started War Paint by developing the four products I've always used myself – concealer, foundation, bronzer and tinted moisturiser. I always knew that one of the prototype products had to be a good concealer for men, because that first time I tried it had had such a huge, transformative effect on me as a teenager struggling with spots.

At the start of War Paint, we had some lovers who got the brand, but we definitely had some haters. I've always stood firm on our simple belief that, as a brand, we want to break down stereotypes and make wearing makeup the norm. All I've ever wanted to do is give men a choice.

'I've always stood firm on our simple belief that, as a brand, we want to break down stereotypes and make wearing makeup the norm. All I've ever wanted to do is give men a choice.'

Get to know Danny

What's your desert island product and why?
Foundation. I've used it every day for the last 20 years to even out my skin, so it's part of my ritual. Or, I'd pack anti-shine powder because it's going to be hot!

What age were you when you first started wearing makeup?
I was about 14 years old. I started getting spots and my sister was like 'here, just try this concealer' and I've used makeup pretty much every day ever since.

What's the average time you take to get ready?
Makeup never really takes me more than five minutes. For my full getting-ready routine – shower included – it's 30–40 minutes. On a bad day, though, it can be a couple of hours if I don't feel confident with how I look. It still happens and I don't think I'll ever be cured completely, but I am learning to deal with it.

How do you de-stress?
Gardening – I'm obsessed. I bought my house seven years ago and the garden looked like an overgrown forest. I got into gardening and find that I just forget about everything when I'm doing it. It's therapeutic. I do have a severe fear of frogs, though, I'm petrified of them.

What are you most proud of?
My two boys, Roman and Rudi. Since I've had my kids, nothing compares to being a dad in any way. They're my inspiration for everything.

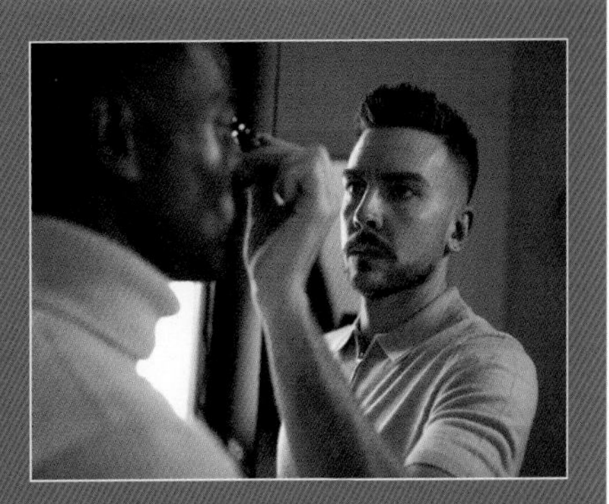

Best piece of advice you've ever been given?
'You don't fail at anything, you only learn.' I'm quite self-critical so it's a great way of thinking for me.

Do you believe in fate?
Yes, I think a lot of the time you make your own luck, but there have been so many things – one email or phone call or bumping into somebody – that have changed everything.

Favourite sport?
I've always been good at sport, but never amazing, which is annoying. I've played semi-professional football, cricket at county level, and I'm down to a six handicap in golf.

Top of your playlist?
Craig David. I prefer his old-school stuff but I love the fact he's reinvented himself. When old-school garage comes on, you're guaranteed to lose me for three hours on the dancefloor.

Ultimate meal?
Anything spicy. For a starter, I would do spicy tom yum soup and for main I'd have a pizza – I always go overboard with toppings like jalapeños.

Dragons' Den

'I just want to start my pitch today by letting you know that I suffer from a mental illness. I suffer really badly with body dysmorphia. I'm telling you this because it's the reason that I founded my brand. My name's Daniel Gray and I'm the founder of War Paint for Men....'

Those were the opening words for my pitch on *Dragons' Den* in front of the five (pretty famous) investors. On camera – and viewed by millions on TV.

I suffer with anxiety and *Dragons' Den* is probably the most nerve-wracking thing I've ever done. Yes, I was absolutely bricking it, but I believed in the brand, 100%. Despite the grilling I got from the Dragons, I was confident about responding to every single question they fired at me. I even did a concealer demo on Theo Paphitis to show them the difference it made.

I talked to the wall

Described as 'one of the best *Dragons' Den* negotiations ever', by the end of my pitch, all five Dragons were competing to invest in War

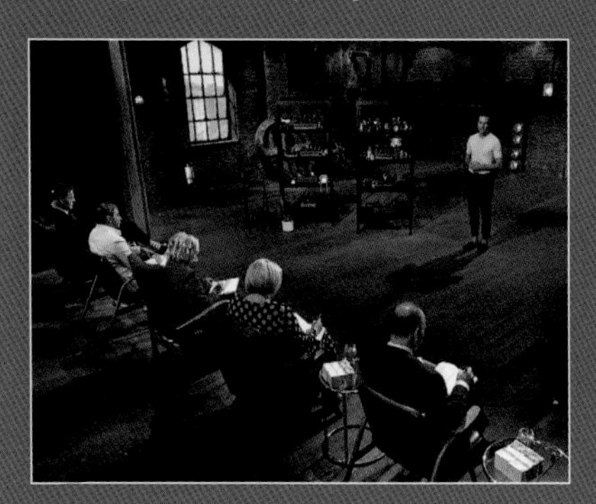

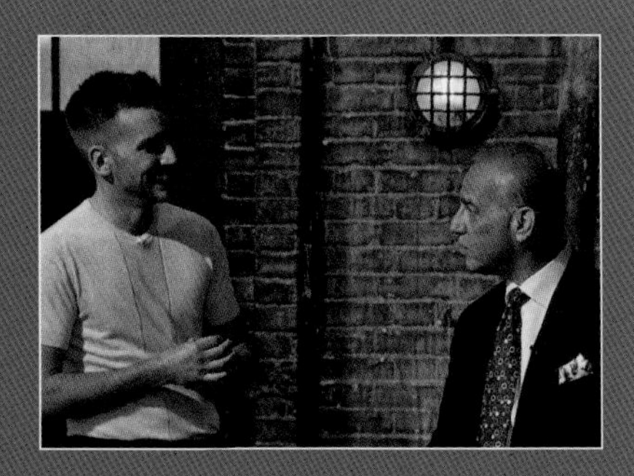

Paint. My head was gone; I was like 'OK, what am I going to do now?' I 'talked to the wall' (if you've watched before, you'll get it) and, after a lot of negotiating, I eventually accepted a joint bid from Tej Lalvani and Peter Jones for £70,000 in return for a 12% stake in the company. Peter Jones said: 'I'm ready to put my War Paint on' and hearing that today still gives me goosebumps. I didn't know what their reaction was going to be and hearing words like that was the biggest relief. I had five investors backing my brand and it felt like it silenced all the doubters.

No deal

After a lot of thought off camera, I eventually rejected the Dragons' offer and decided to go it alone. Some of you might have seen the episode on BBC2, or heard about the buzz it caused, but getting that reaction from not only the Dragons but also the viewers once the episode aired gave me that reassurance that I really was on to something with War Paint – and the market for men's makeup. Even though we're not working with the Dragons, we've had an amazing ride and the plan all worked out in the end. It was honestly the most amazing experience of my life and something I'm so grateful for. Plus, it gave men's makeup a platform on prime time TV.

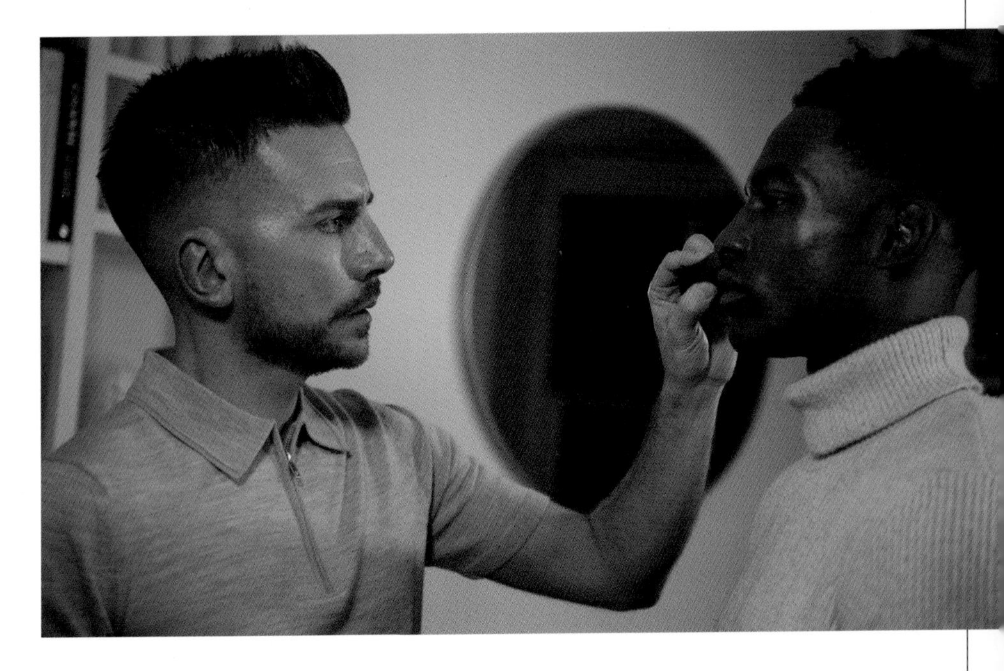

War Paint has changed my life forever, in ways I could never have imagined. We're so much more than a cosmetics line. We're a brand leading the way in the revolution that is men's makeup.

Why makeup?

These days, a lot of guys are cool with spending hundreds of pounds a year on moisturisers and skincare to make their skin look good. So my thinking has always been, why not extend that to makeup to deal with the dark circles and cover blemishes? For me, it's a no-brainer.

I know that a lot of men don't understand makeup, or find it complicated (trust me, it isn't). That's why a massive part of War Paint is education (in simple man speak), from online tutorials to this manual you're reading right now. No flowery language, no bullsh*t and no set rules.

For me, learning to use makeup has been a massive confidence booster at times when I've been at an all-time low. I'm not saying that makeup is a miracle potion for low self-esteem (if we had that, we'd bottle it), but using makeup has really helped me to manage my body dysmorphic disorder and feel good about myself.

I'm not trying to change the world, or save people's lives, but I know there are so many guys out there who are struggling with stuff that they don't need to. Whether it's makeup, or something else, there are tools out there to help you get through it.

I hope War Paint – and this book – will open up doors for men everywhere to wear makeup with confidence and shout about it.

'For me, makeup has been a massive confidence booster at times when I've been at an all-time low.'

About War Paint

Men's makeup is not a new concept. Check out the next history section for the lowdown on that. But men's makeup that's mainstream and sitting on a counter dedicated solely to guys? That's War Paint.

You may not be used to seeing the words 'men' and 'makeup' in the same sentence (not until you've read this book, anyway), but that's because there's never been anything like this for guys before.

Our research shows that men arc reluctant to go to a women's counter to buy makeup products, but put men's makeup in a retail department space designed for guys and everything changes. War Paint is helping to break down stereotypes about who buys makeup, who wears makeup and how you apply it. It's not rocket science (trust us).

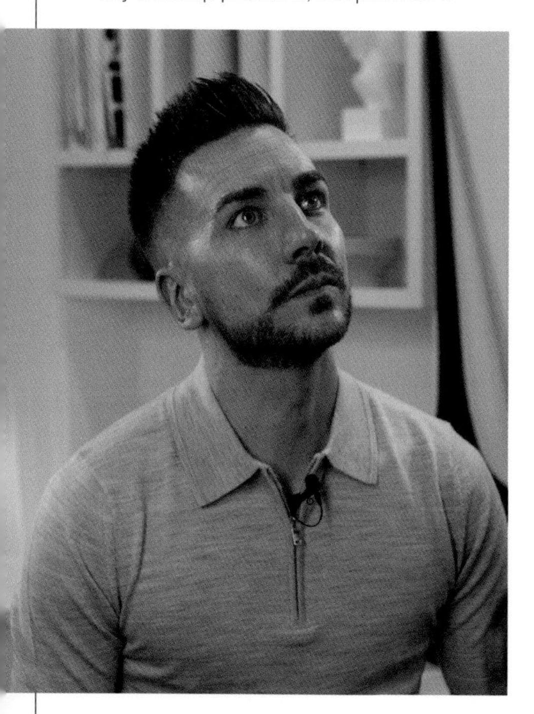

War Paint products

War Paint is a cosmetic brand that's been formulated and designed for men. Our foundation is called foundation, and our concealer is called concealer – there was never any debate about that when we started out in 2018. We don't want to hide what our products are – we just want to educate men about what the products do, and the (pretty massive) benefits you can get from makeup.

Why put up with dark circles every morning when you don't have to? The truth is, just like women, we also struggle with skin concerns, whether it's a spot that refuses to budge or unexplained redness. The key is knowing that you can do something about it with makeup.

War Paint products are specifically made with a guy's skin in mind because we deserve to feel good about ourselves, too. Makeup is just a tool to make that happen.

'We don't want to hide what our products are – we just want to educate men on what the products do, and the (pretty massive) benefits you can get from makeup.'

Our key War Paint makeup:

Concealer
Great for hiding dark circles, spots, scars and blemishes.

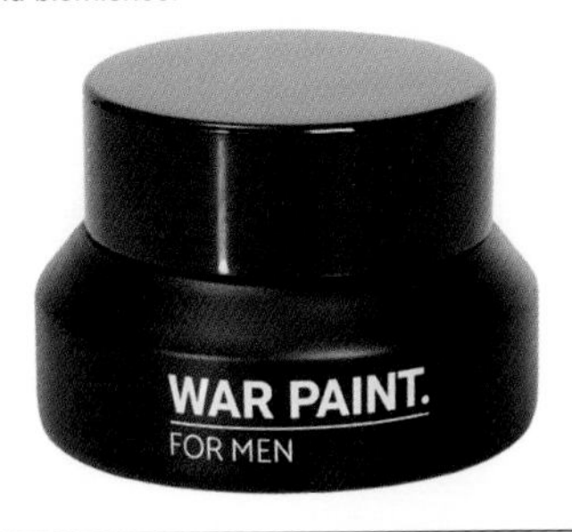

Primer
Helps keep your makeup in place and gives your skin an even finish.

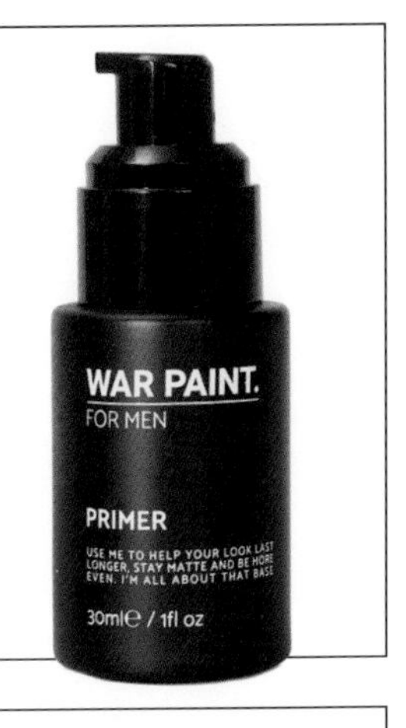

Tinted moisturiser
Gives you light coverage for a more natural look.

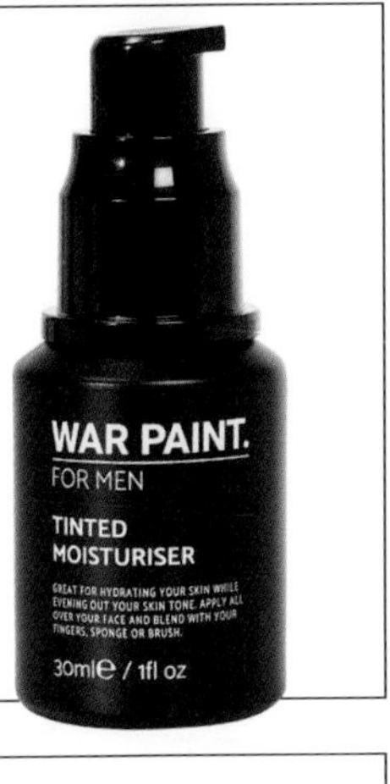

Bronzer
Gives you the instant appearance of natural, bronzed skin.

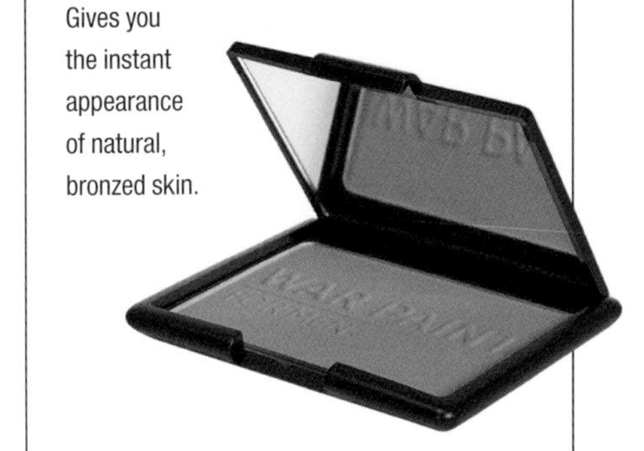

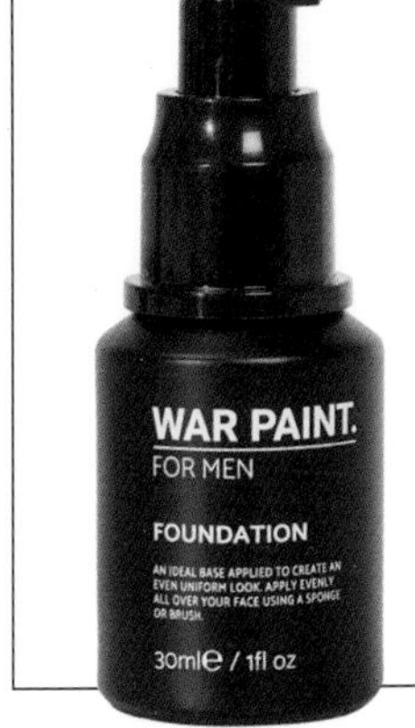

Foundation
Use as a base to give your skin an even, uniform look.

Anti-shine
A transparent powder to help eliminate unwanted oil, shine and sweat.

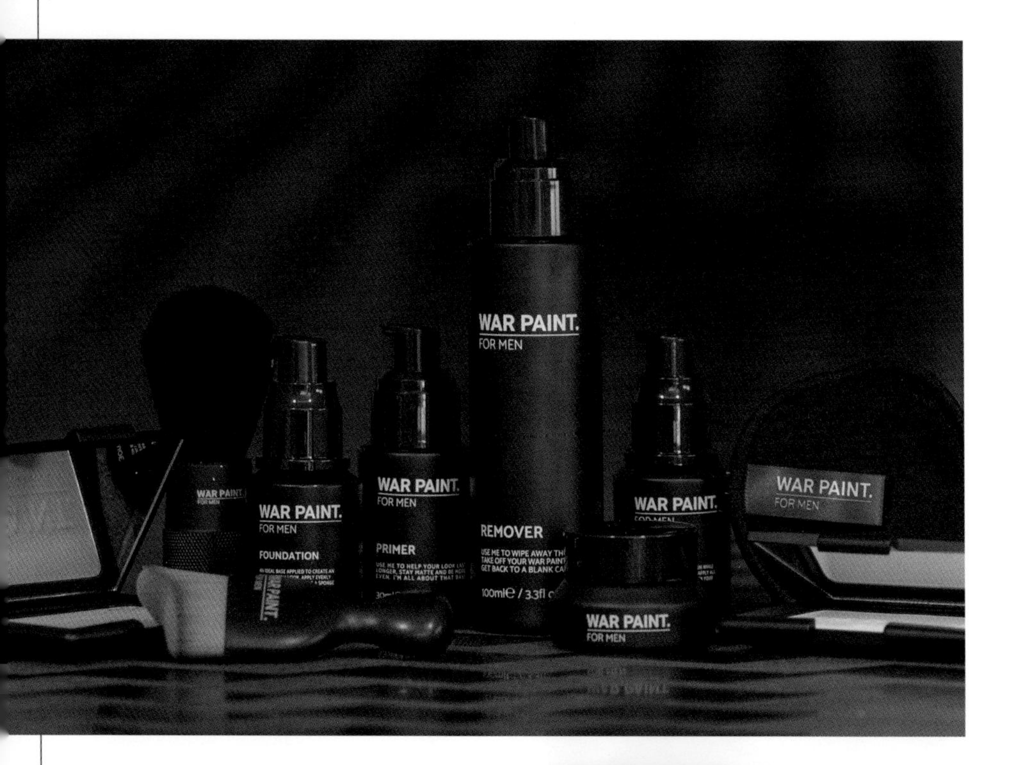

Changing perceptions

Yes, we're a brand selling makeup, but War Paint has also become a strong advocate for mental health. We're changing perceptions and challenging masculine stereotypes every single day. When I first started the brand, nobody was talking about men's makeup and now, two years on, we've been in more than 500 press articles globally. We're bringing awareness that it's OK to use products to make you look (and feel) good.

Men have always been using makeup in the background, but War Paint brings makeup for men to the forefront. We get it, there's still a stigma surrounding men wearing cosmetics. We want that to stop, because there is nothing to be ashamed about. Men's makeup is here to stay. Full stop.

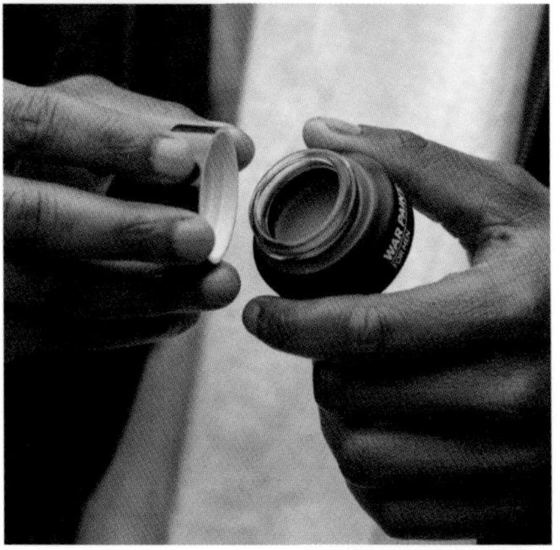

'Men have always been using makeup in the background, but War Paint brings makeup for men to the forefront.'

The War Paint timeline

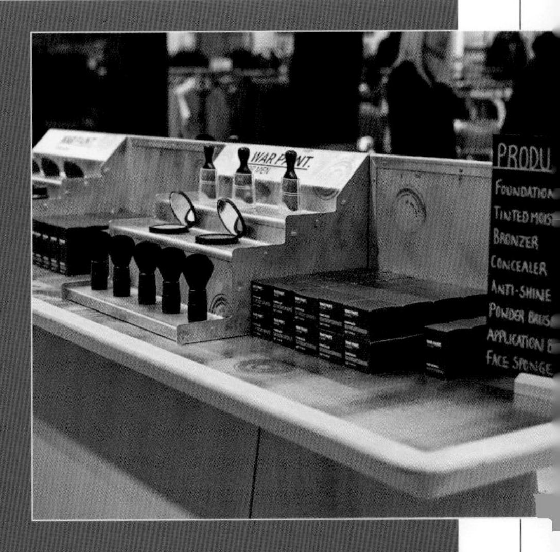

November 2018:
War Paint launches online
In the first six months, the brand sells 15,000 products.

May 2019:
War Paint goes viral
In just 24 hours, 'War Paint' gets 8 million views online.

September 2019:
War Paint airs on *Dragons' Den*
All five Dragons want to invest in the brand.

November 2019:
War Paint is one
In its first year, War Paint sells over 50,000 products – more than five times as many as I suggested I would achieve in my pitch to the Dragons.

December 2019:
War Paint hits the high street
War Paint becomes the first all-male makeup brand concession in UK major department stores, including Harvey Nichols and John Lewis.

February 2020:
War Paint goes stateside
War Paint opens its dedicated US warehouse.

March 2020:
War Paint expands retail
The brand confirms more major retail partners, including John Bell & Croyden, Reiss and Mr Porter.

June 2020:
War Paint takes off
War Paint partners with Virgin Atlantic to become the first men's makeup brand available in the air.

July 2020:
War Paint goes global
The brand launches in Japan, as well as Brown Thomas and Arnotts in Ireland. War Paint now sells in more than 80 countries around the world.

August 2020:
War Paint does football
War Paint signs a deal to become the official training shirt sponsors for Championship football club Norwich City FC.

January 2021:
War Paint in Sephora
War Paint launches in multinational retailer Sephora.

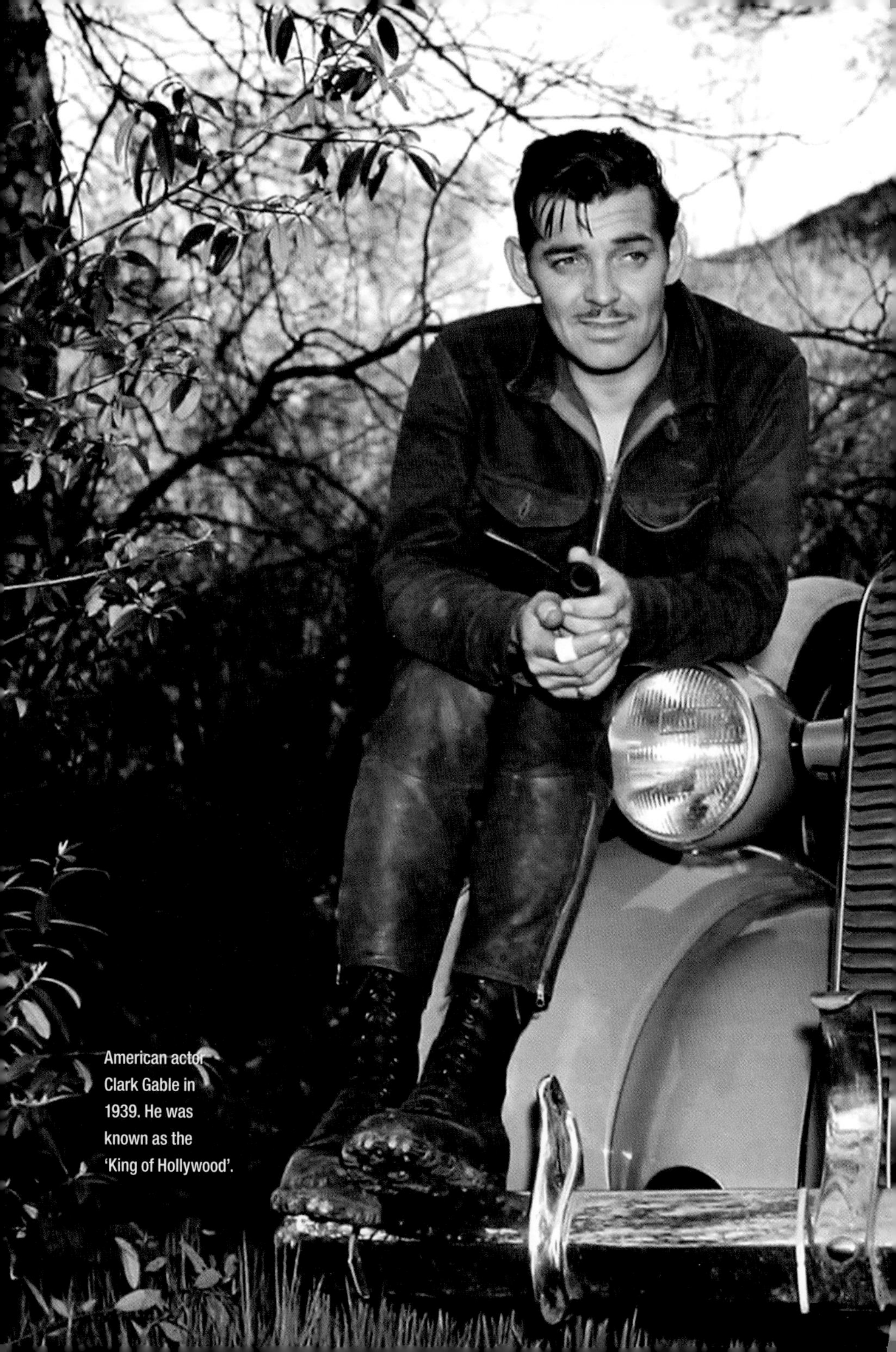

American actor Clark Gable in 1939. He was known as the 'King of Hollywood'.

Chapter 2

The History of Men's Makeup

Men's makeup has evolved massively through the years. From 4000 BC when men used to line their eyes with kohl, to today when guys wear a bit of concealer to boost their confidence, we chart the use of makeup from then to now.

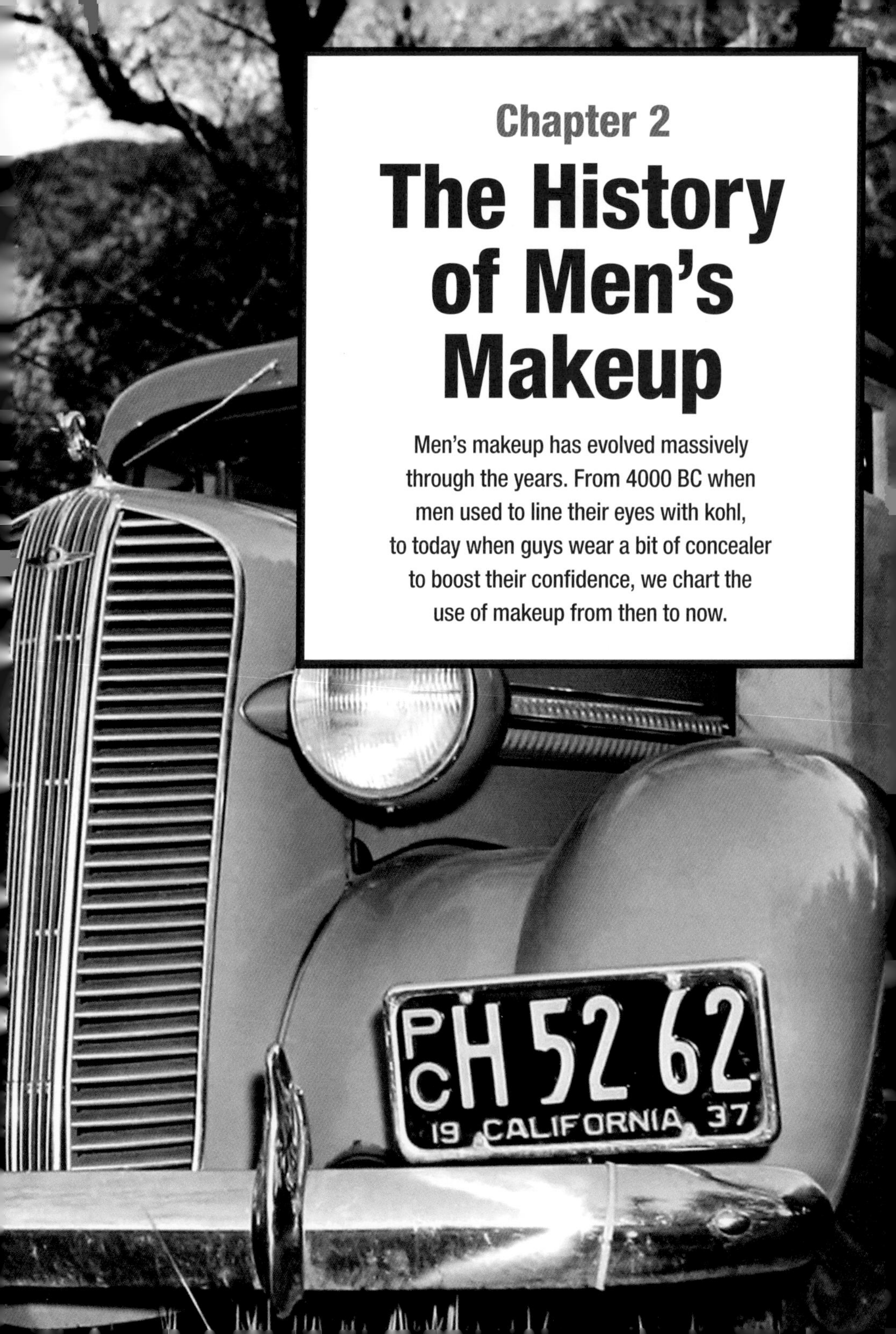

Coming full circle

You might be surprised to know that makeup for men is not a new thing. In fact, it's now come full circle in being completely normal – but it's taken centuries to get there. Here's how it happened.

The origins of men's makeup

The origins of men wearing makeup is thought to date right back to ancient Egyptian culture, as early as 4000 BC. No, pharaohs didn't apply foundation for a night out at the pyramids, but they did use black pigment to create elaborate cat-eye designs, which are documented on the etchings and paintings that you see on ancient tomb walls.

There doesn't seem to be any difference between how men and women used make up in Ancient Egypt, and although it was the nobility who enjoyed the most expensive products, it is thought that the lower classes also had their own, more economical versions. By 2650BC, Egyptian men were using a whole host of 'products' – black kohl eyeliner, green eye pigment created using malachite, and lip and cheek stains made from red ochre. Application 'tools' came in the form of smoothed wood or bone. Makeup wasn't worn to look good, but for practical, medicinal and magic reasons. For instance, the distinct almond-shaped eye represented the Eye of Horus, which was believed to be a symbol of protection and good health.

↑ Eye of Horus, which was replicated in the style of Egyptian makeup.

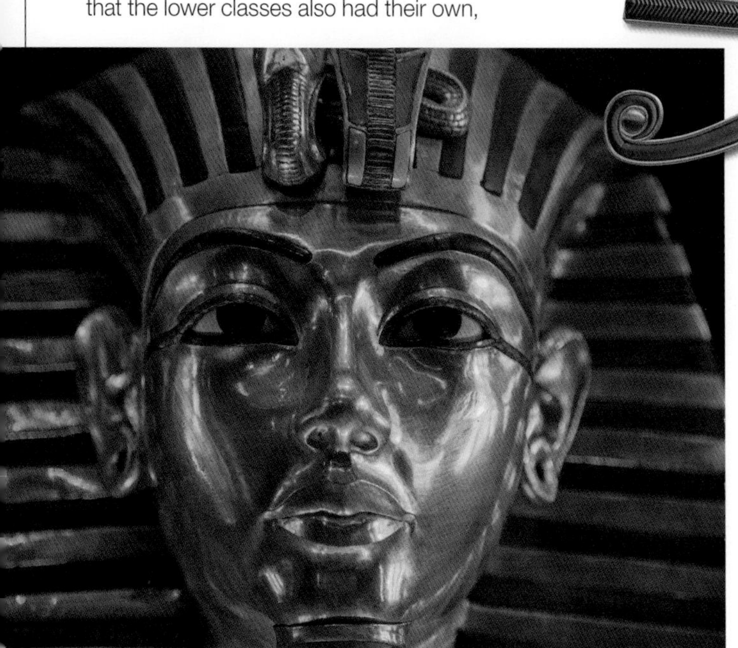

← Pharaoh Tutankhamun's mask, with ancient guyliner.

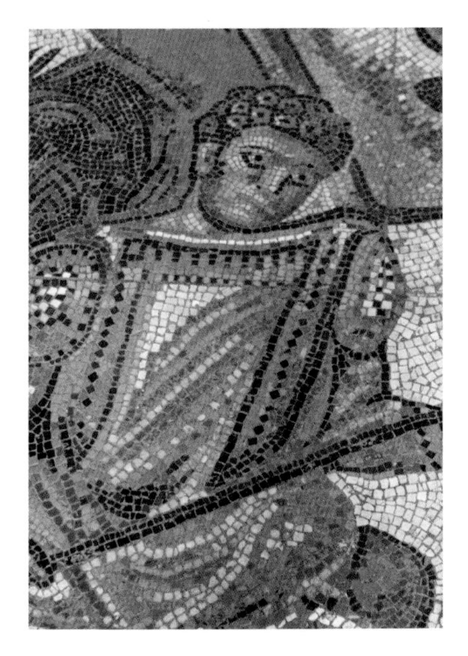

Imperial Roman mosaic with a touch of rouge on the cheekbones.

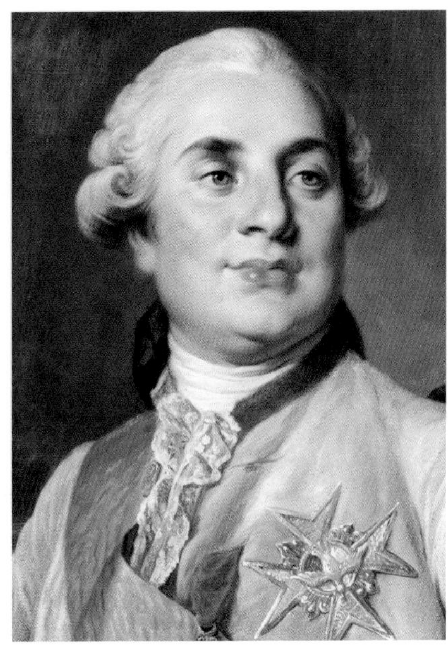

King Louis XVI's pale complexion was a sign of status.

How makeup evolved

Fast-forward to the 1st century AD and red pigment was still around in Ancient Rome – but used in a different way. Some Roman men lightened their complexion with powder and added rouge to their cheeks, like some kind of blush prototype. We might have high-tech, vegan-friendly product formulations today (count yourself lucky), but the 'rouge' used on cheeks back then was often a mix of pig fat and blood.

While we're using a dash of bronzer for an instant tan, the 'in' skin colour for men during the early modern era (1500–1800) was palest white. Why? It suggested wealth and idleness rather than having to work in the fields and getting sunburnt, so a ghostly white, powdered face became a sign of status throughout the 17th and 18th centuries. Unfortunately, this was also the era when said white face makeup was often made from lead, which, unsurprisingly, caused health implications or, worse, induced premature death.

Monarchy and makeup

In 18th-century France, King Louis XVI set the aristocratic beauty agenda for extravagant makeup and big wigs. Men of the royal court also painted on beauty spots for instant status. In the absence of a dab of concealer, some beauty spots were strategically worn to cover signs of disease, such as smallpox.

Timeline of Men's Makeup

This simple timeline charts how men have used makeup through the ages.

4000BC
Ancient Egyptians use dark pigments to rock a bold line in eye make up.

1st century AD
In ancient Rome, men lighten their complexion with powder and add red pigment to cheeks.

16th century
Super-powdered white faces are all the rage and Elizabethan men use tactics like beauty spots to conceal blemishes and signs of disease.

19th century
Queen Victoria rules that makeup is 'vulgar' and wearing heavy makeup becomes a) highly unfashionable and b) frowned on for men.

1930s
Modern moviemaking in Hollywood means there are dedicated hair and makeup trailers for male stars, such as Clark Gable.

1970s
Music icons such as David Bowie and Prince put the limelight on cosmetics for men with bold stage makeup.

1984
Culture Club's Boy George releases Boy George: Fashion and Make-Up Book to help his fans nail '80s makeup looks.

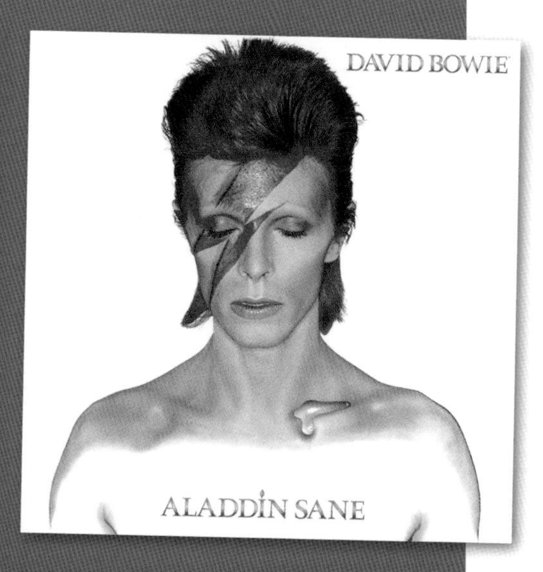

↑ Electrifying makeup on David Bowie for his iconic 1973 Aladdin Sane album cover.

2000s
Guyliner transitions from punk-rock rebellion to sex symbols on the red carpet. See poster boy looks on Jared Leto and Brandon Flowers for reference.

2008
Beauty brands start to release targeted makeup for men. Yves Saint Laurent launches the male version of its bestselling Touche Éclat.

2009
Movie star Zac Efron wears foundation and makes headlines.

2017+
The YouTube generation take the internet by storm and lift the taboo for everyday makeup for men.

Girls only?

Makeup has been seen as a 'women-only' thing for generations (until now, that is), so when did the no-make-up-for-men shift happen? Turns out it wasn't until the mid-1800s when painted faces – on both men and women – were dubbed 'vulgar' and male grooming quickly faded into the background.

At that time, Queen Victoria deemed cosmetics 'the devil's work', and the Church of England agreed, giving all cosmetics some seriously bad PR. The youthful Queen Victoria didn't like makeup and ruled that only whores should wear it. Only male actors were exempt from the rule and encouraged to perform in drag to play female roles, since it was strictly forbidden for females to be actors. In general, though, men wearing makeup was considered taboo and the idea stuck.

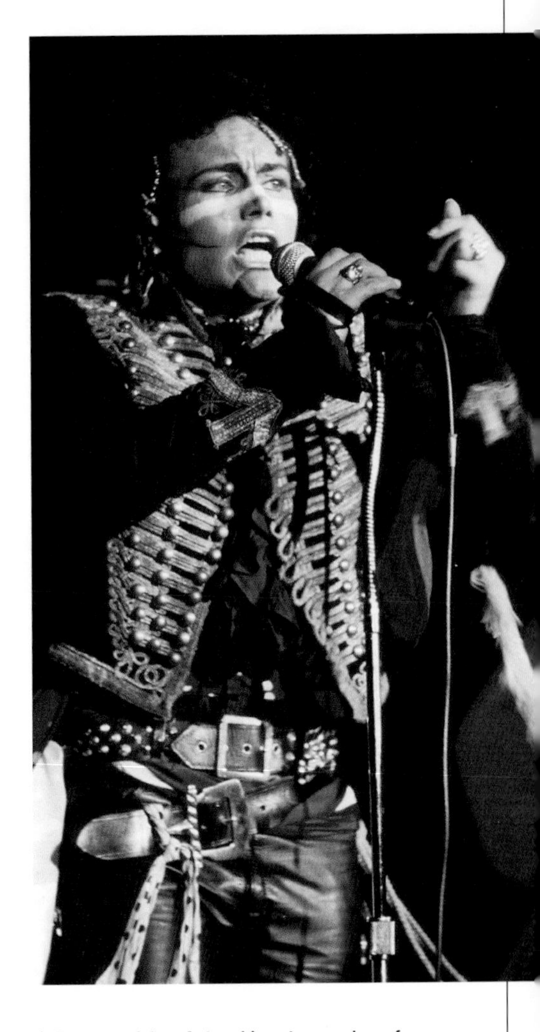

Frontman Adam Ant rocking stage makeup for a 1981 Adam and the Ants performance in London.

A return to men's makeup

After going into a long retirement (thanks, Queen Vic), makeup for men finally started to make its comeback in popular culture in the last third of the 20th century thanks to music legends such as David Bowie, Prince and Adam Ant, who brought it firmly into the limelight in the 1970s and 1980s. Even then, though, makeup for men was hardly mainstream, and when worn by the stars, it was always bold and exaggerated. Who can forget that iconic lightning bolt on Bowie's 1973 *Aladdin Sane* album cover?

In the early 2000s, the Egyptian-inspired eyeliner made a return with the concept of rock stars wearing 'guyliner', aka heavily kohled eyes. It's only in the last few years, though, that makeup for men has shifted from larger-than-life stage makeup to the natural, everyday looks that now feature on YouTube tutorials and Insta demos. Seeing blokes on social media who teach you to apply concealer to cover up dark circles, or use foundation for a fresher-faced look, has helped remove the stigma of makeup for men for future generations, for good.

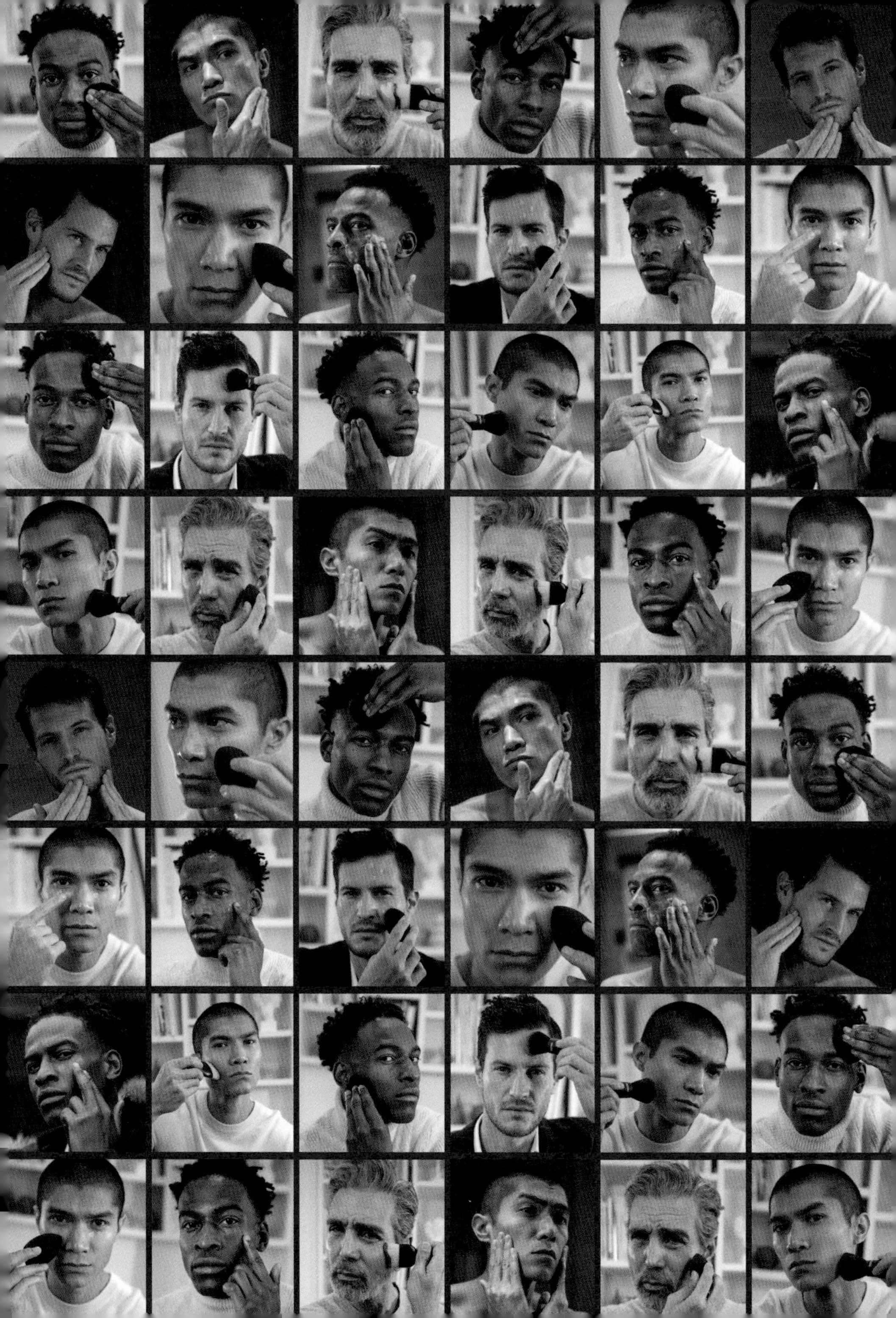

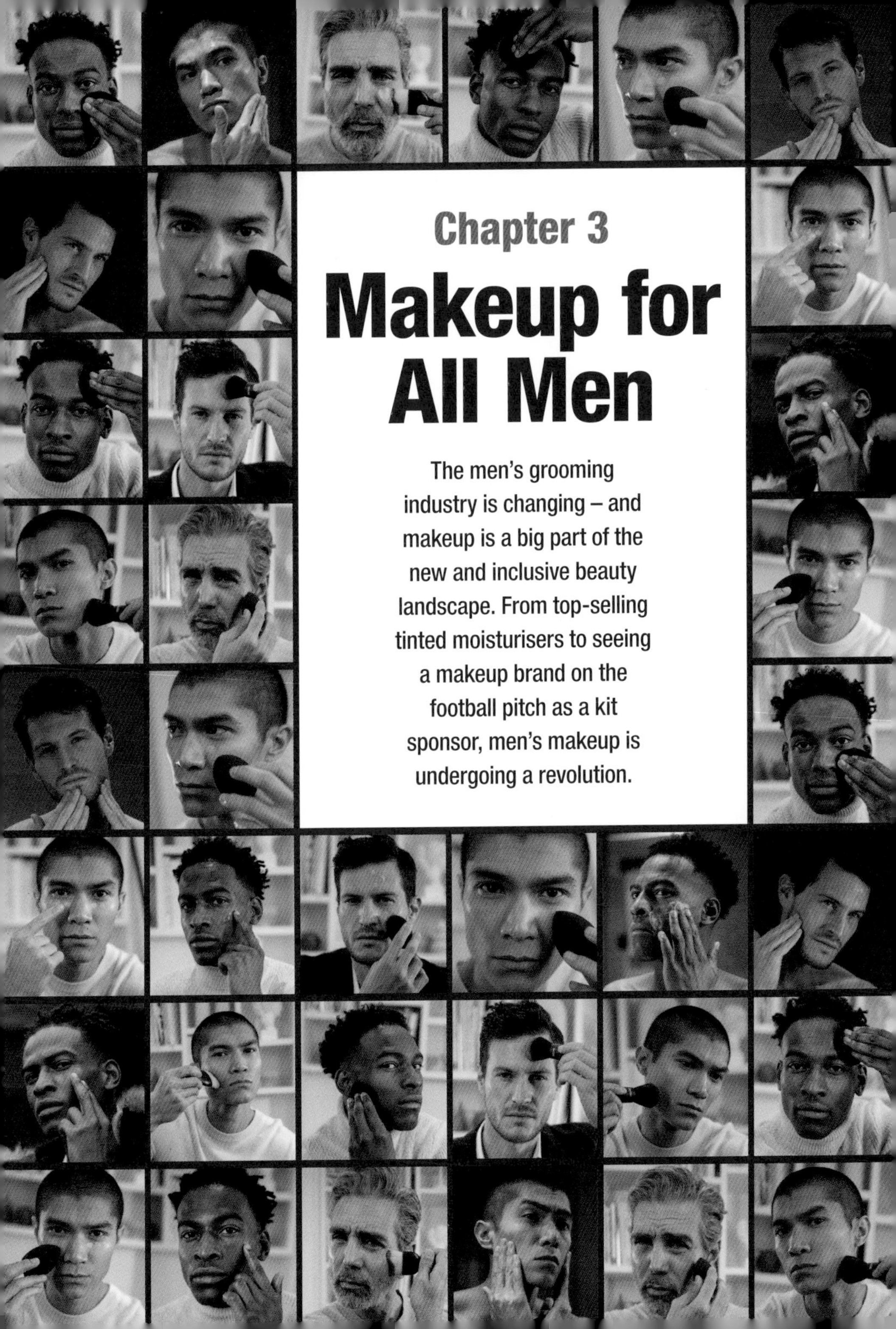

Chapter 3

Makeup for All Men

The men's grooming industry is changing – and makeup is a big part of the new and inclusive beauty landscape. From top-selling tinted moisturisers to seeing a makeup brand on the football pitch as a kit sponsor, men's makeup is undergoing a revolution.

Men's makeup revolution

Remember a time when people used to make fun of guys who used moisturiser? Because who would want hydrated skin, right (spot the sarcasm there)? In previous generations, the idea of men using moisturiser seemed pretty radical, but then celebrities like David Beckham started fronting major grooming campaigns in the late 1990s and normalised being a bloke and looking after yourself with products.

Fast-forward to today and men's beauty is a multi-million pound industry and makeup is just another way for us guys to improve our look. You apply product to make your skin look good – simple. This shift in the way we view men's beauty – we can also call it 'grooming' if you prefer – is happening globally. In recent years, the boundaries of men's beauty have been pushed so we're seeing a more inclusive industry than ever before.

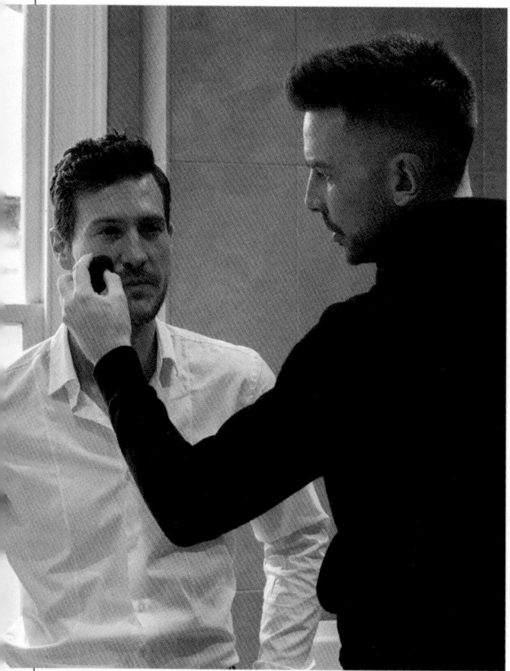

Men's grooming is the fastest growing segment of the beauty market, and was valued at £500 million in the UK alone in 2019.

June 2019 data from market analyst The NPD Group

Makeup: the numbers

Let's be real here: we're genuinely ecstatic that makeup for men is being talked about (it's about time), but this isn't some passing beauty trend like those weird fish spa pedicures that became a five-minute wonder. As far as we're concerned, makeup for men is a movement that's here to stay and the statistics prove it. Over half (56%) of men in the USA admitted to wearing some sort of cosmetic such as foundation, concealer or tinted moisturiser at least once in 2018, according to a survey by Euromonitor.

Over in the UK, one in 30 (3%) of men now wear makeup, according to a recent 2019 YouGov survey* – and that's just the guys who admit it.... Going on the UK population of 67.9 million (of which men make up about half), if you do the maths, that's more than a million guys who regularly wear makeup. Some forecasters predict that within five years, one in four men will use some type of makeup product.

* YouGov British men and makeup survey, February 2019

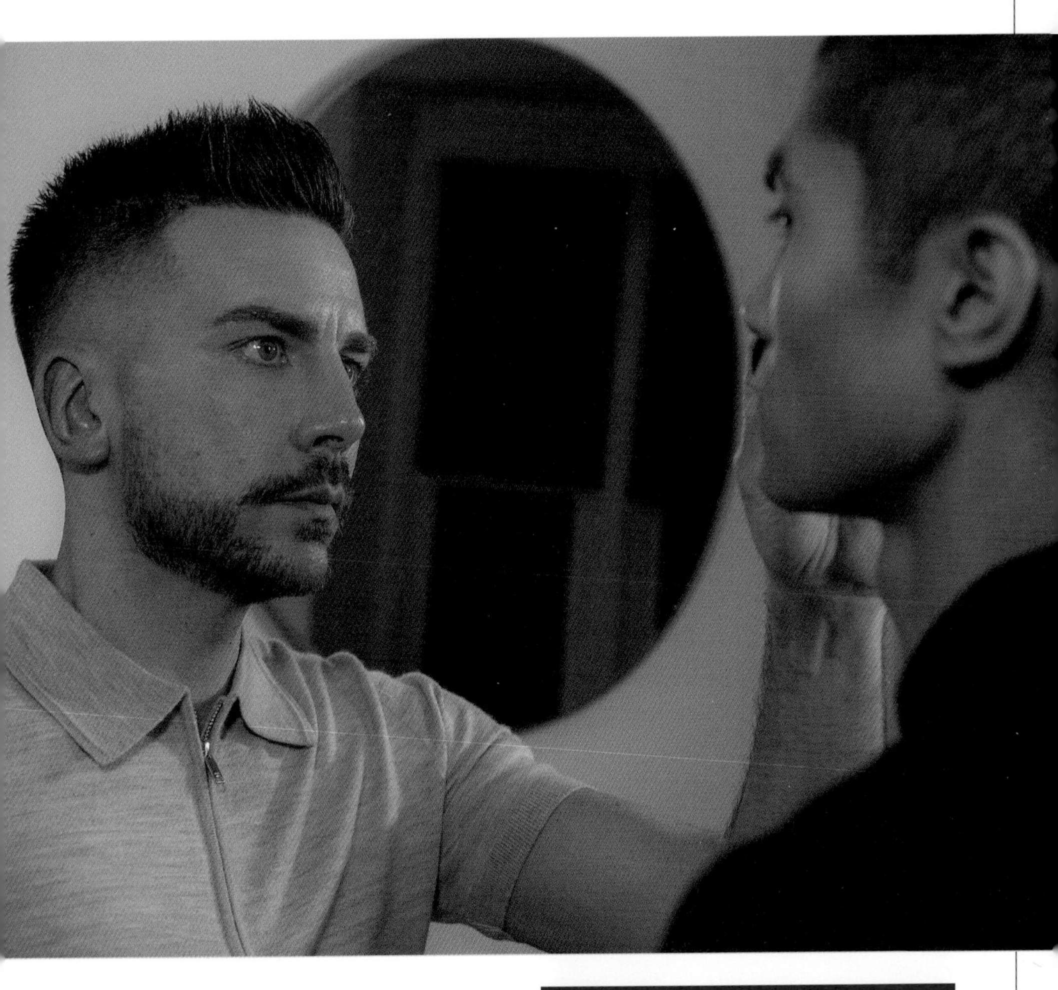

What's in our shopping carts?

The days of boshing on a bit of moisturiser and hoping for the best are over. Whether it's a quick-fix concealer to cover a spot, or something more regular like a tinted moisturiser to even out skin tone every day, men are wising up to makeup products that make a difference. Like their high-tech skincare, the Asia-Pacific market is a step ahead when it comes to makeup and is one of the fastest-growing regions for men's grooming and cosmetic product use, according to Coresight Research.

Reasons men cited for wearing makeup

- 13% wear makeup to hide blemishes.
- 11% wear makeup to feel good.
- 9% wear makeup to help change a feature on their face.
- 8% wear makeup to boost their confidence.
- 4% wear makeup to look professional.

YouGov British Men and Makeup survey, February 2019

Iman Bokolo, at Cosmetify (www.cosmetify.com)

'Today's society promotes a bigger acceptance of different sexualities, races, genders and abilities – more so now than ever before. This means that gender norms are finally being challenged, which in turn helps men to feel less pressure when indulging in what was once a typically "feminine" ritual.

'With brands such as War Paint releasing products like bronzers and concealers that cater to men, I think the men's beauty industry is progressing to become more inclusive. Like women, men have faced pressures within society for their physical appearances and the launch of men's makeup highlights the spike in men's interest in the beauty industry in recent years.'

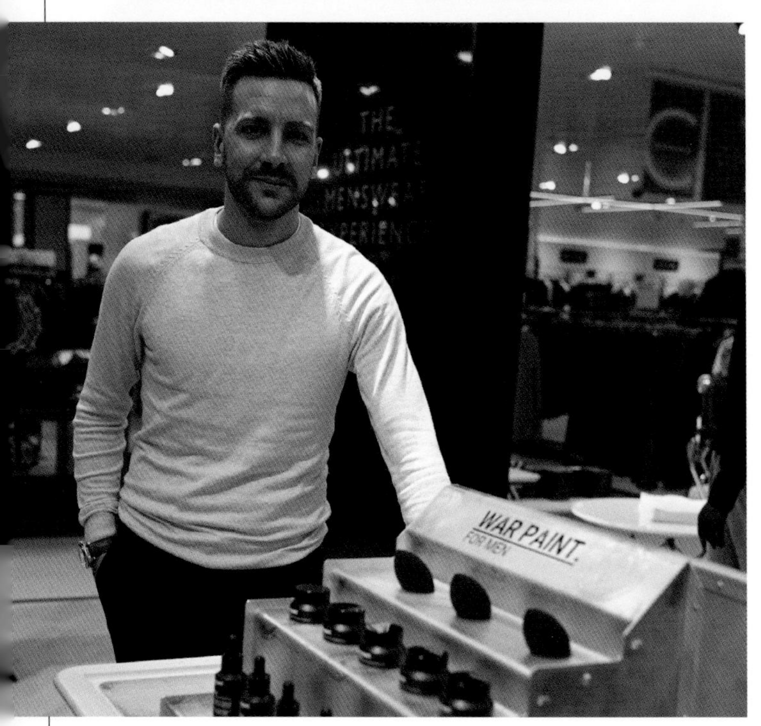

← A world first. Danny at the War Paint counter in John Lewis's flagship on London's Oxford Street - the first ever all-male makeup brand to have a concession in a department store.

In China, current supply isn't able to meet the high demand for men's makeup products.

This growing waiting list for men's makeup is part of a global grooming industry that's expected to top $81.2 billion in 2024, according to Statista. On the Cosmetify platform, War Paint – and the top-seller, tinted moisturiser – sits alongside global giants Clinique and Tom Ford as one of the three most popular men's makeup brands. When War Paint set up a trial retail stand in London's Oxford Street in 2019, its male customers exceeded demand and bought out a month's worth of stock in one week. The bestseller? Concealer.

THE LOWDOWN:
Women buying War Paint

Believe it or not, a lot of women buy our products too (for the men in their lives to use) – 44% vs 56% men. Why? It tells us that guys have confided in their partner that they feel like shit about their blemishes or dark circles under their eyes, and their other half is doing something about it.

Who's buying War Paint?

As makeup for men is being talked about more and more in mainstream media, as the founder of War Paint, I'm often asked about whom my 'target audience' is. People assume our typical customer is a tanned 22-year-old who goes down the gym every day and out on the pull every night, but the reality is pretty different. When I first trialled War Paint on a retail counter in 2019, I had customers ranging from 14-year-old boys to 75-year-old men. There is no demographic for men's makeup, it's exactly the same as the market for women.

There's the guy in his 40s who wants to smooth out his wrinkles at work so he looks more youthful on his work Zoom calls, there's the new dad in his 30s who wants to lose the dark circles from too many sleepless nights, and then there's the teenager who's struggling to leave the house because of his acne. Every guy has their own story about why they want to use makeup. Our online figures show that 33% of our customers are aged 18–35, 35% fit into the 35–50 category, and 32% are over 50, so it's a pretty even split. Regardless of the date of birth on your driving licence, our ethos has always been makeup for *all* men, regardless of age, skin tone or sexual orientation.

It's always been important for us to cater for as many skin tones as we can with the shade range that we have. We offer as many dark shades as we do fair – that was key for us – and it's something that the makeup industry as a whole needs to address.

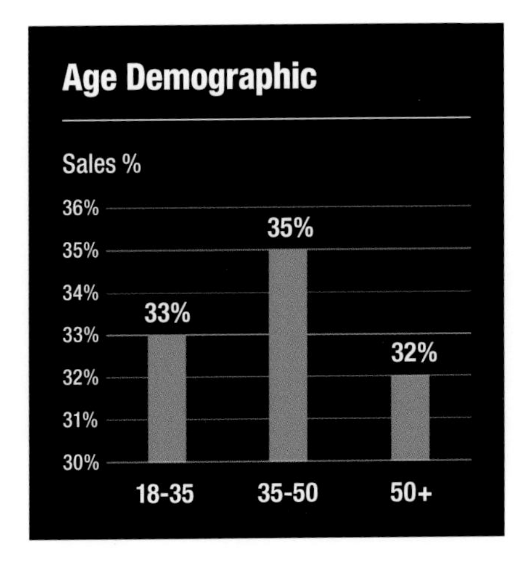

Football focus: Norwich City FC

In a few short years, War Paint as a brand has evolved so much, but one of the things I'm proudest of is sponsoring Norwich City FC for the 2020/21 season. This wasn't about footballers putting on foundation because they're paid to do it (and it being really fake) – it was more about breaking the stigma and signalling that it's OK to put on products to feel good.

We get it: a men's makeup brand and a football club might not seem like the most obvious link-up, but the partnership grew from a shared commitment to open up about men's mental health. Both brands want to challenge stereotypes and break down the boundaries that can affect guys every day.

At War Paint, we've always wanted to stir up the conversation about both men's makeup and mental health to normalise them; to put something like concealer on the agenda for the kind of banter you'd have with your best mates on a Friday night in the pub. Doing something like partnering with a football team was a way for guys to take notice and talk about makeup, whether they agree with it or not....

We knew we were going to get some football fans saying 'that's ridiculous, footballers and fans don't wear makeup', but you'll also get other people going 'oh, well that's cool'. And that's what we need to do to make this normal – break the taboo. We've had hundreds of supportive messages from people all over the world who are behind the sponsorship. Of course, we've had the opposite

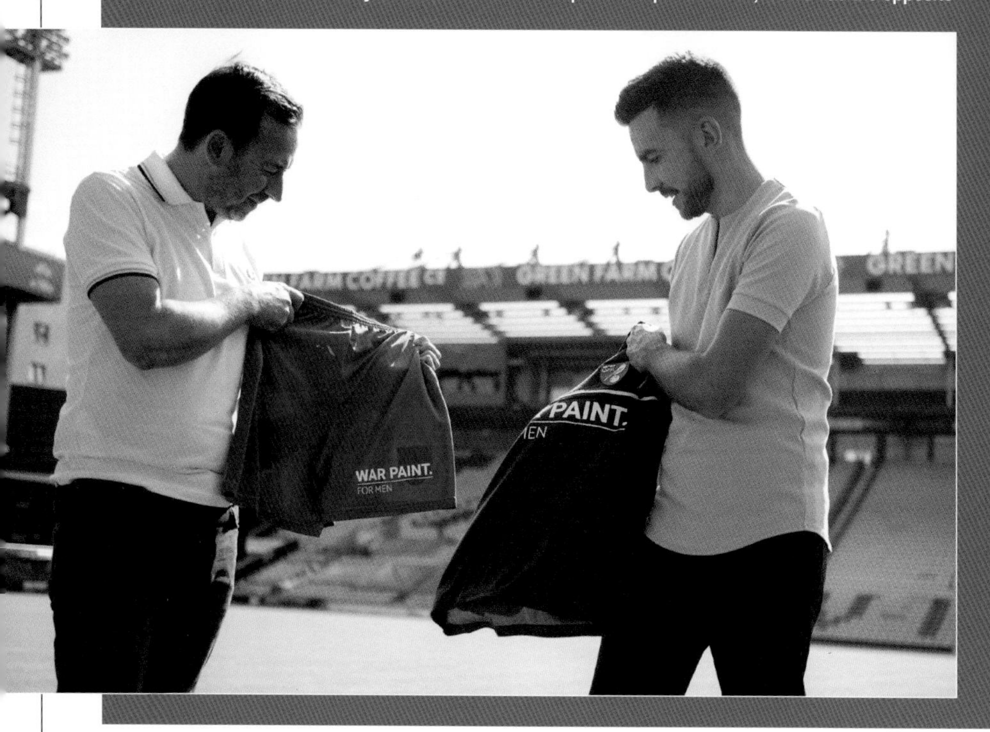

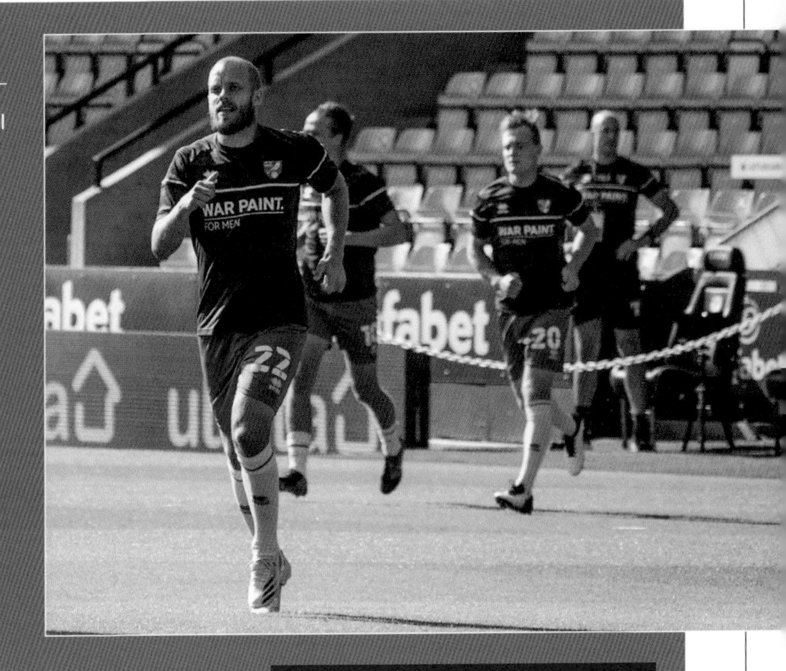

➔ Norwich City football players on the pitch in War Paint training kit.

➹ Danny with Matt Lumb, War Paint CEO, checking out the War Paint sponsored Norwich City FC kit at Carrow Road.

reaction, too, with haters saying 'we play like women, now we're going to look like women'.

Ultimately, there are a lot of guys who are going to benefit from seeing War Paint on Norwich FC kit. They'll see their favourite player wearing our brand on the team shirt and think 'oh, OK, I'll give it a go', because it's validation. I honestly believe that we'll look back in ten years' time and say 'I can't believe that was ever a thing: men questioning makeup'. We need to keep talking and raising awareness so we get that long-term shift in attitude that sticks.

The partnership with Norwich City FC has also led on to some amazing link-ups with major personalities and thought leaders around challenging stereotypes. Stephen Fry saw what we were doing with makeup and as advocates for men's mental health and wanted to get involved because he believes in our message. We hope others do, too – regardless of what football team you support.

THE LOWDOWN:

Makeup vs football

What the fans see: the 2020/21 sponsorship puts War Paint's branding on the back of the main kit shorts, on the away kit, as the main logo on training kits, and on advertising boards around the Carrow Road pitch.

Our link-up also includes a commitment from both War Paint and Norwich FC to donate a percentage of the sponsorship funds back into Norwich City FC's official charity partner, the Community Sports Foundation, so everyone's a winner.

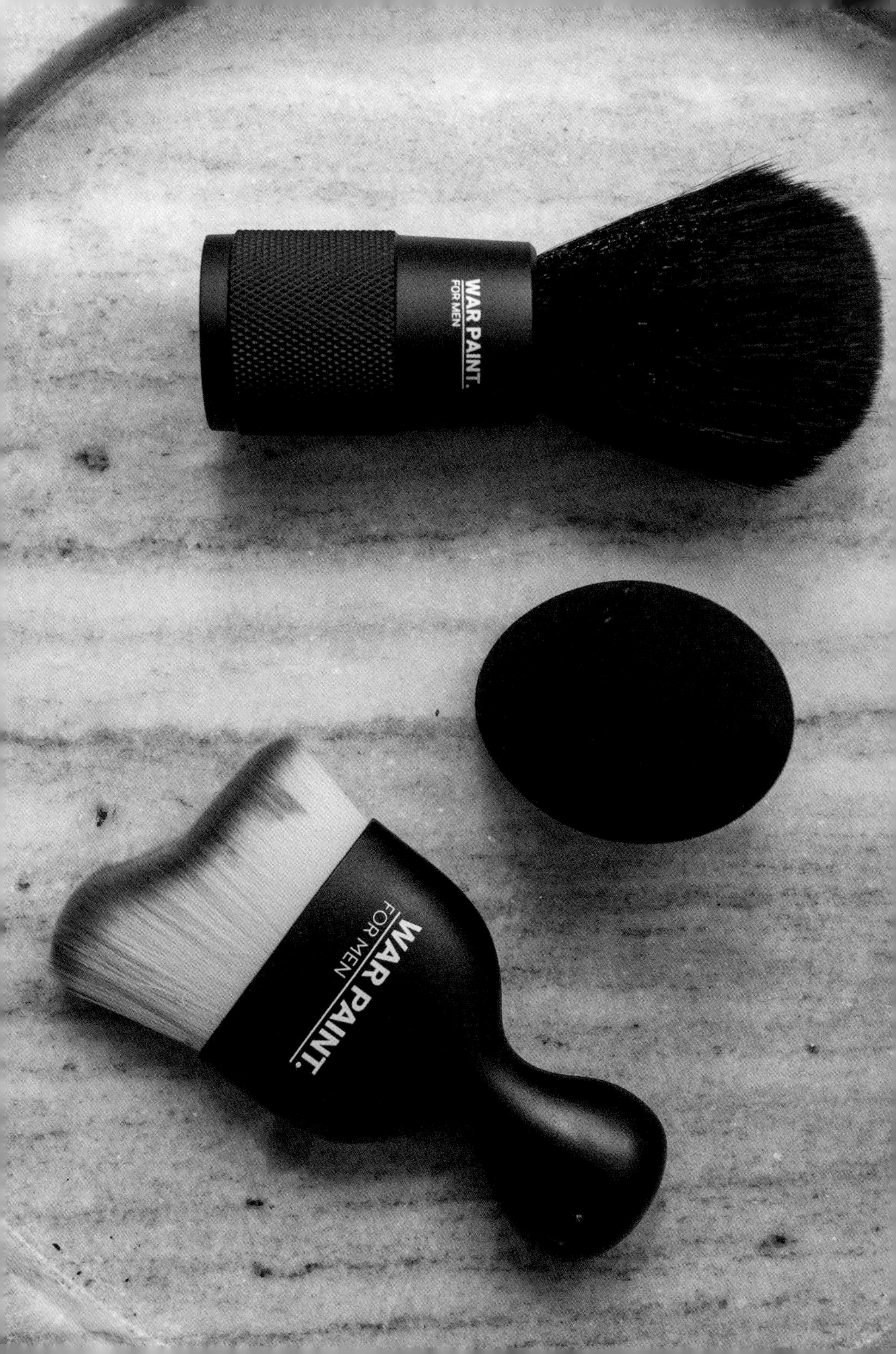
WAR PAINT.
FOR MEN
WAR PAINT.
FOR MEN

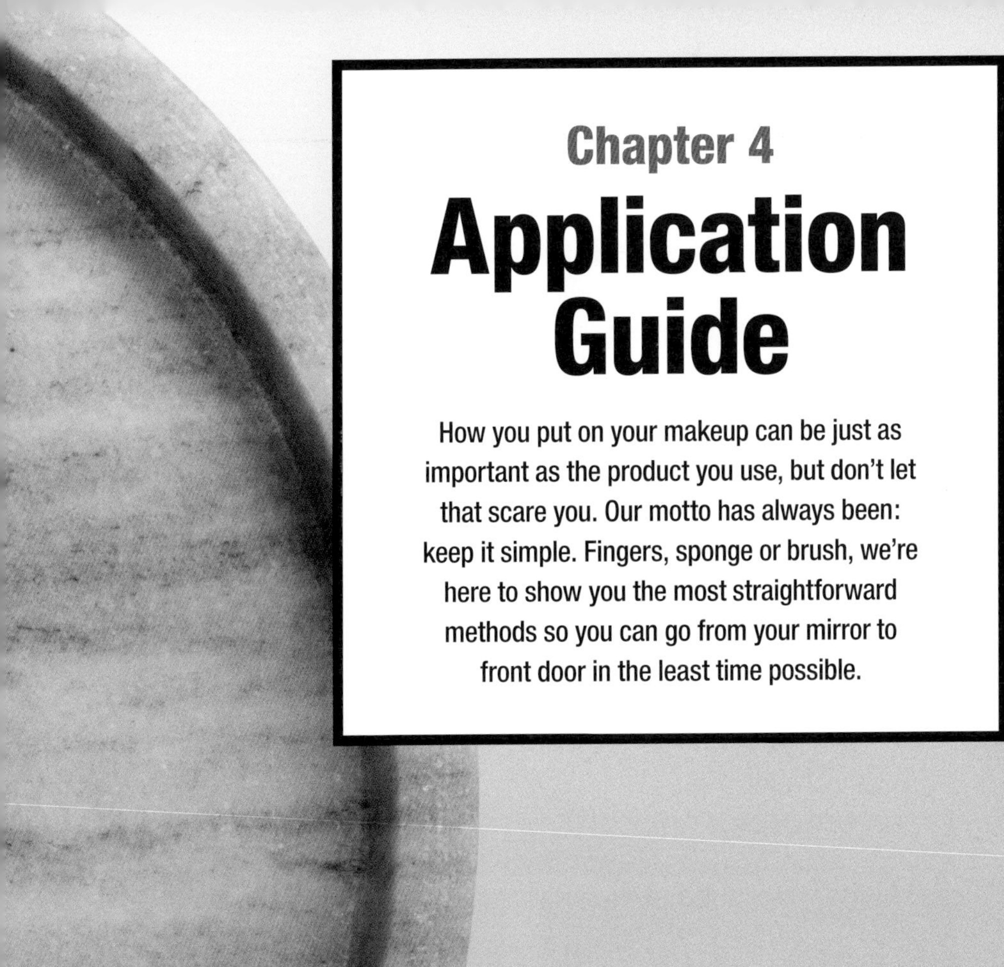

Chapter 4

Application Guide

How you put on your makeup can be just as important as the product you use, but don't let that scare you. Our motto has always been: keep it simple. Fingers, sponge or brush, we're here to show you the most straightforward methods so you can go from your mirror to front door in the least time possible.

The tool kit

There's one rule to follow when it comes to men's makeup: there are no rules. It's that simple. And the same applies to your application tools. Whether you use your fingertips or tools, you can still achieve the same natural finish. Professional makeup artists use different application methods so it's all about finding the one that works best for you and your skin.

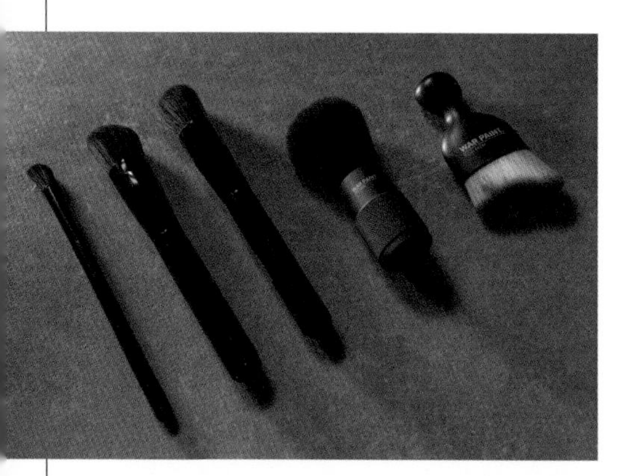

Brushes

Some of you may prefer to apply product with brushes. It's certainly best to apply powder products in this way as they give good, even coverage – something that is not so easy to achieve with fingertips. Smaller brushes can make it easier to be more precise if you're using something like concealer.

The size and density of your brush depends on what you're applying so it's always good to find the right brush for the

How to clean tools

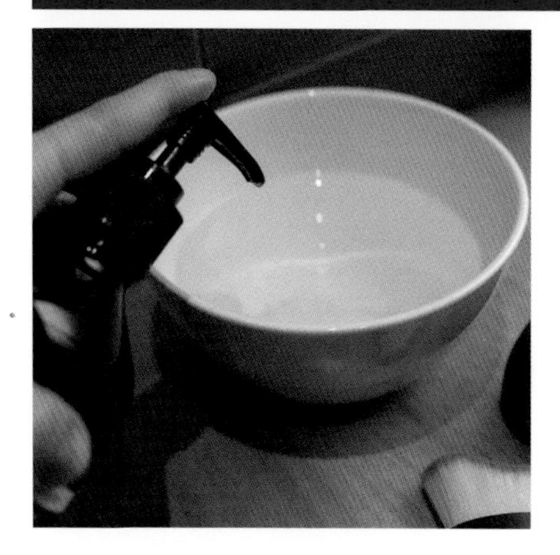

1 Fill a bowl with warm water and add a little gentle shampoo for natural hair bristles or washing-up liquid for synthetics/sponges.

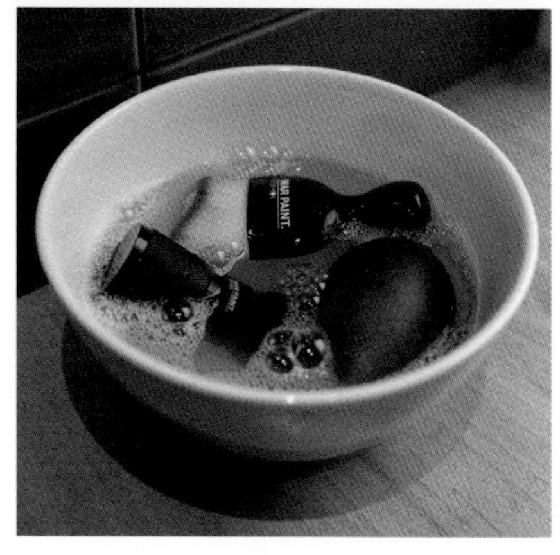

2 Leave to soak and then swirl the brushes/squeeze the sponge in the water to lift out any dirt.

right task. A large powder brush with a softer texture is great for finishing your look (see Chapter 7). At the other end of the spectrum, if you're using a brush to apply liquid products then a denser brush is your go-to option. If you've made the call that brushes are for you, it's a good idea to have two to four good-quality brushes in your kit.

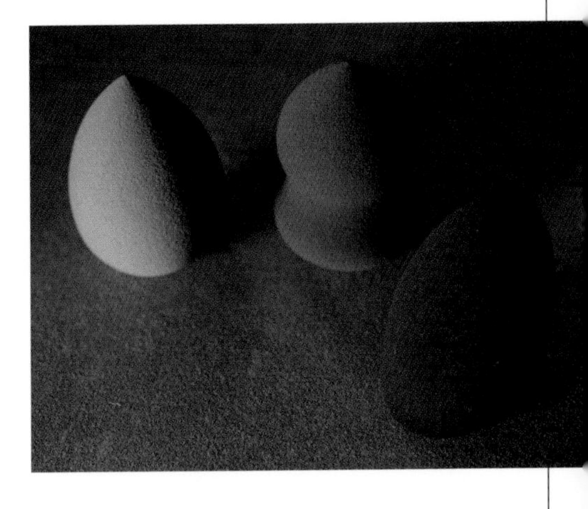

Sponges

A bit of a multitasker, you can use a face sponge to blend concealer, foundation and tinted moisturiser. You'll be pleased to know there aren't as many variations of makeup sponges as there are brushes. Egg shape (or teardrop) sponges are perfect for blending out makeup on larger and smaller areas, such as the creases of your nose. A sponge with a flat, angled side is especially handy for extra precision and smoothing makeup.

Sponges can be used wet or dry. Used damp, they're less likely to produce the telltale streaks that brushes can sometimes leave behind.

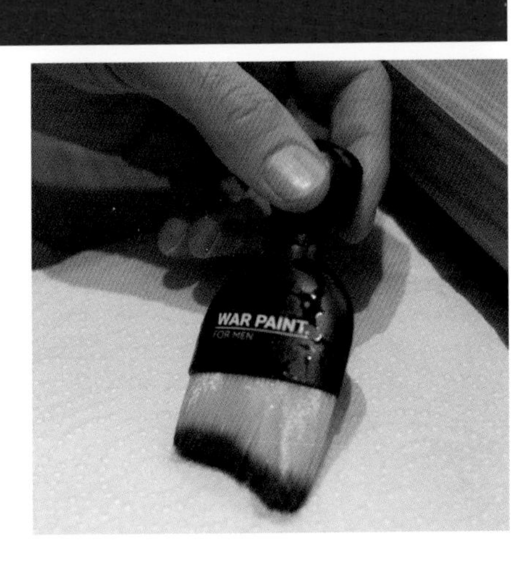

3 Rinse well, blot with paper towels, then lay flat and leave until completely dry.

Get into the habit of regular tool maintenance to keep your kit in check. If you don't wash your brushes and sponges regularly, you'll be inviting bacteria and other nasties on to your face (yup, we're talking sweat, dead skin cells and other facial hair dirt) that could cause breakouts. Aim to deep-clean your brushes at least once a month to keep them in good nick. Because it's mega-absorbent, try to give your makeup sponge a quick rinse after each use and ideally replace it every three months.

Application methods

When it comes to primer, foundation and concealer, you can use a ton of different application techniques. They all do the same job, but in different ways. If you're fairly new to makeup, start off with the finger method, for the greatest level of control. You can then go on to experiment with tools such as brushes and sponges if you want to achieve a different finish.

The finger method

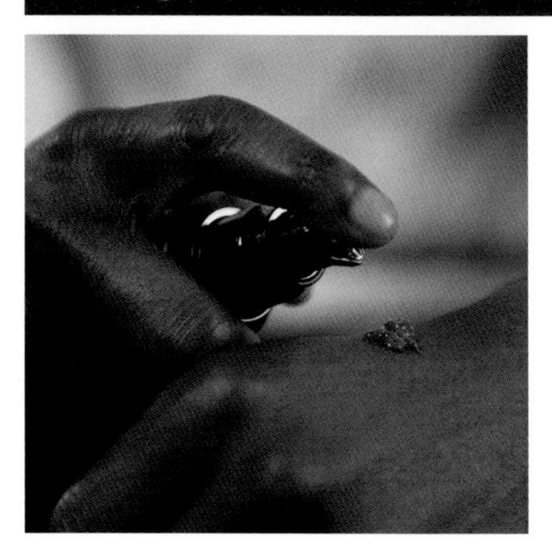

1 Apply a small amount of product on to the back of your hand or fingertip. You can always add more product, but it's harder to remove too much.

The sponge method

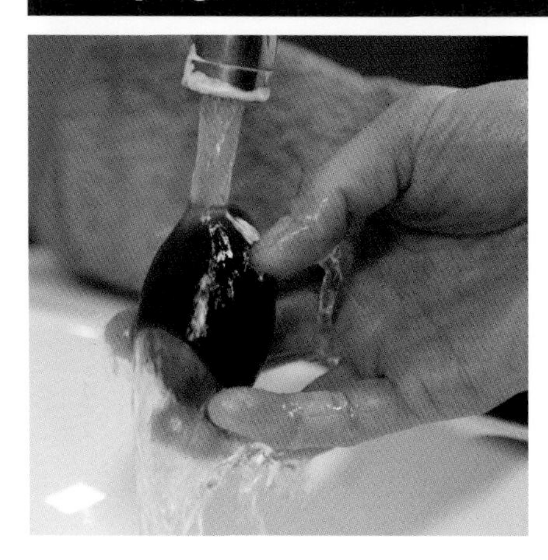

1 Dampen your sponge before using it. Run it under a tap so it expands and then squeeze out any excess water.

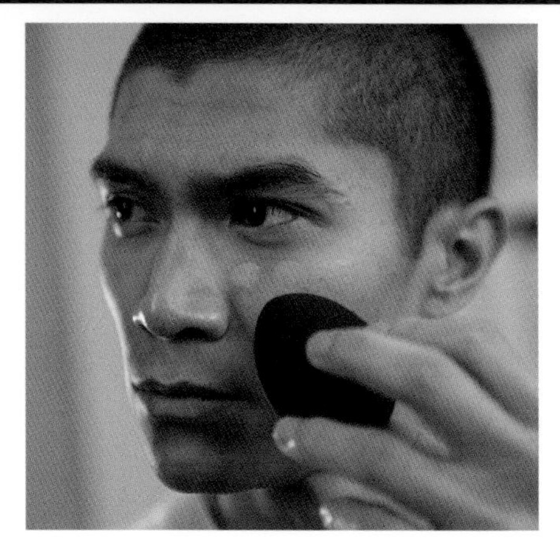

2 Dot the product lightly on to your face and then blend with the damp sponge.

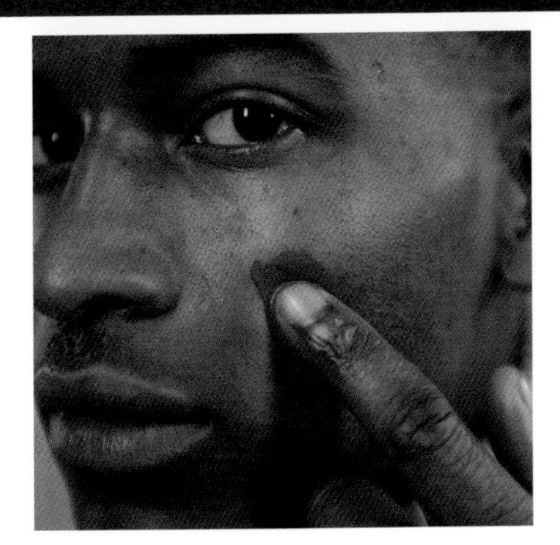

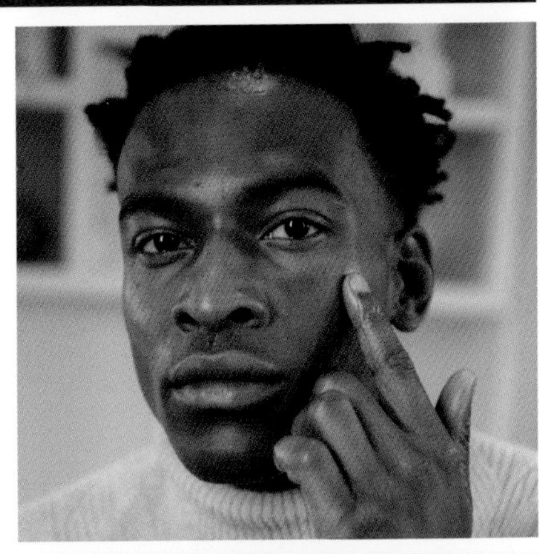

2 Using a fingertip, apply the product to your face. Lightly tap the product into the desired area until it's fully blended in.

Scan to watch the
'finger method'
step-by-step video

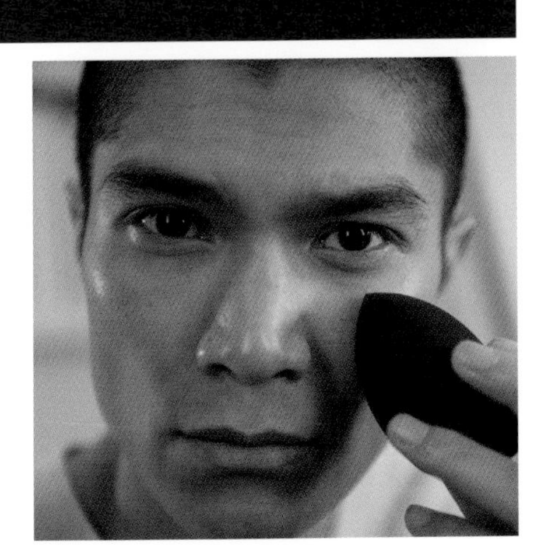

3 Dab the sponge around your face, pushing the product in to blend evenly.

Tip

Not sure how to clean your sponge? Leave it soaking in warm water and then use the back of a tablespoon to squeeze out any excess makeup and dirt.

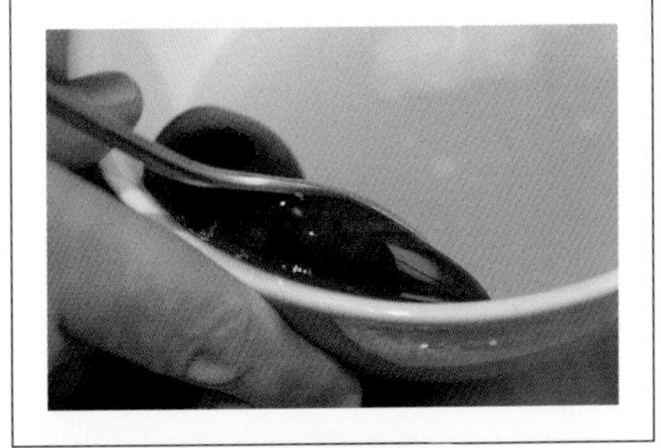

Scan to watch the
'sponge method'
step-by-step video

The brush method (liquids)

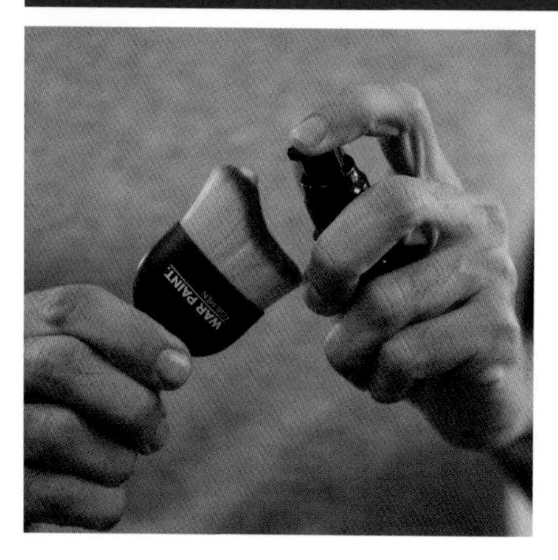

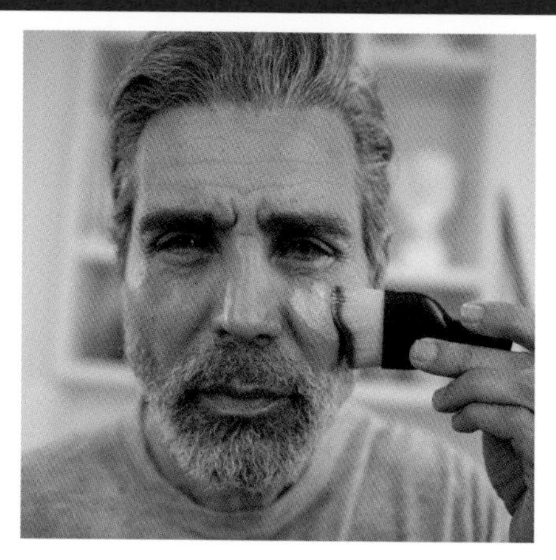

1 Dot the product on to the brush hairs. Start with a small amount so you can build up to the level of coverage you want.

2 Blend the product across the face without applying too much pressure.

The brush method (powders)

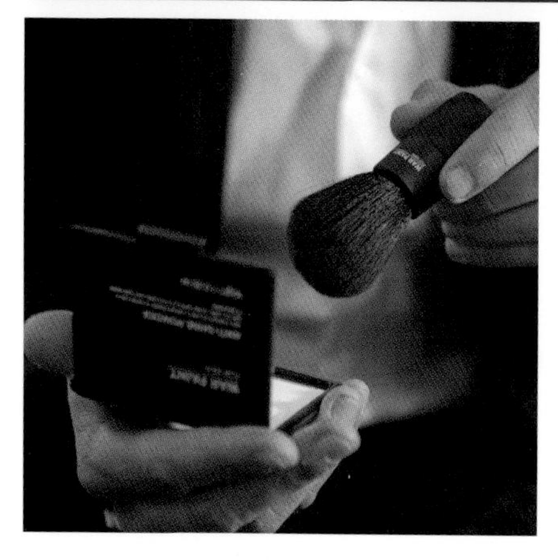

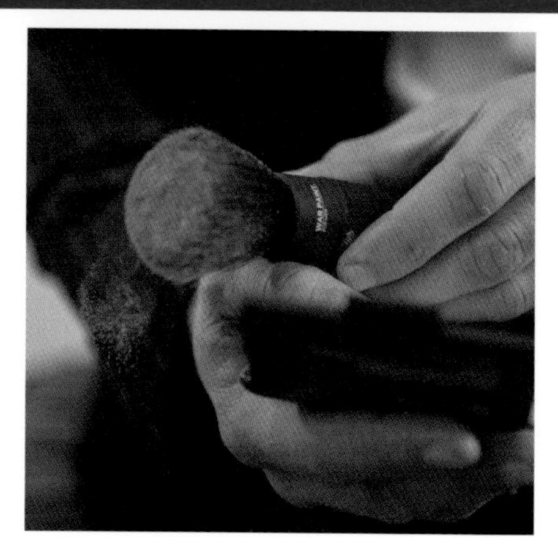

1 Lightly sweep a powder brush over the product.

2 Tap or blow off any excess powder.

3 Continue to use light, sweeping motions until the product is undetectable on your face.

Tip

Don't get too hung up on how to apply your products – there is no right or wrong way. Scan our QR code tutorials to see the how-tos in action.

Scan to watch the **'brush method (liquid)'** step-by-step video

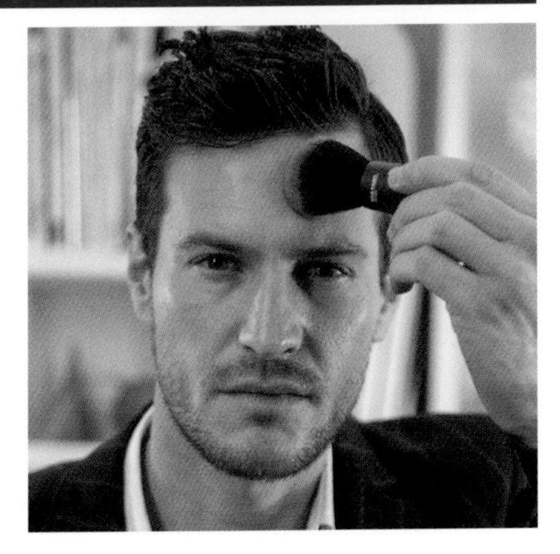

3 Use light, sweeping motions on your face to apply the product evenly.

Do and don't

✓ Do apply your products in natural daylight if you can. It not only gives you the most accurate reflection of your face, but it's also easier to see when something isn't fully blended.

✗ Don't use dirty tools (yup, your fingertips included). Try to get into the habit of washing your tools regularly to avoid breakouts.

Scan to watch the **'brush method (powder)'** step-by-step video

The application guide

We've mapped out your makeup so you don't have to. From prep to removal, here's the War Paint lowdown on key products for men – and the tools you can use to apply them.

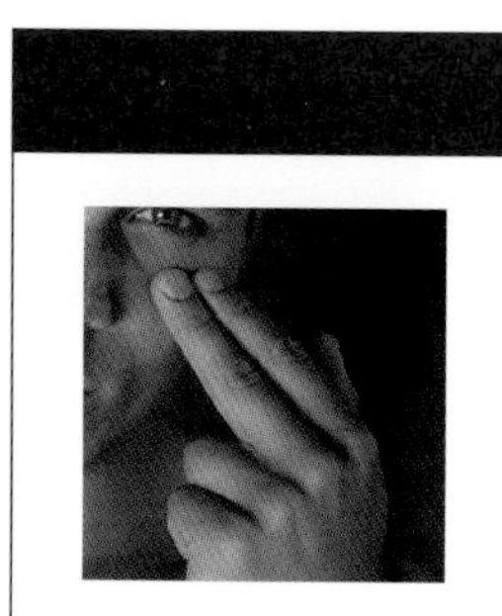

Fingers

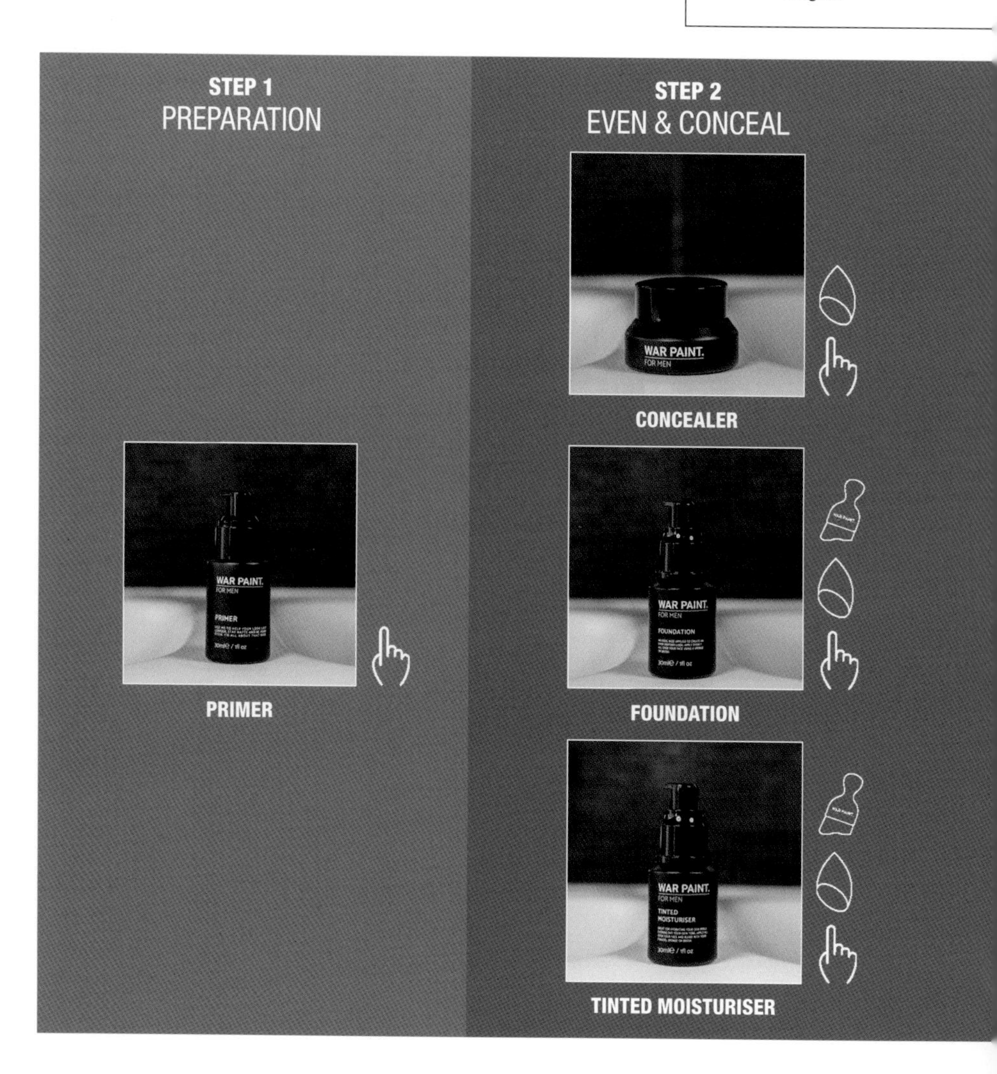

Application tools

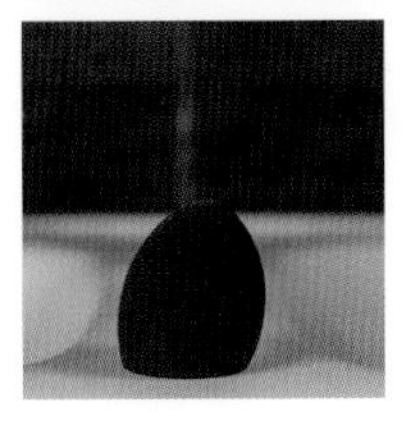
Sponge

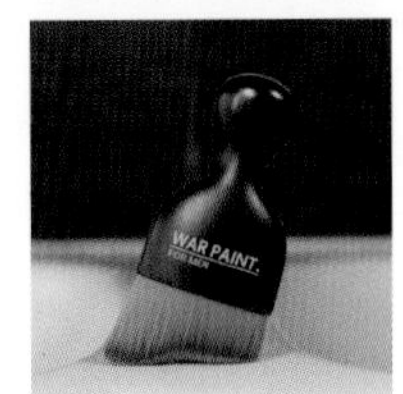

Application brush

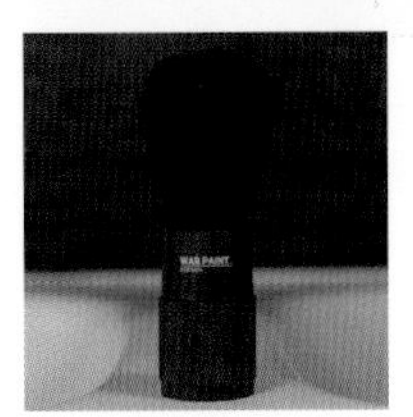
Metal powder brush

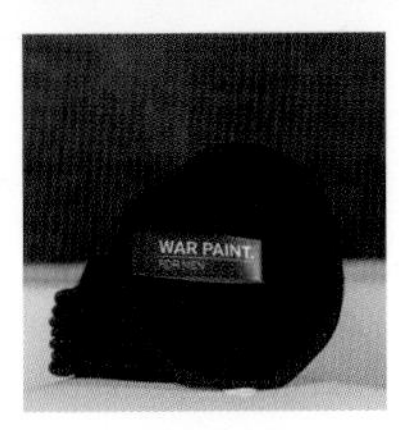

Reusable bamboo pads

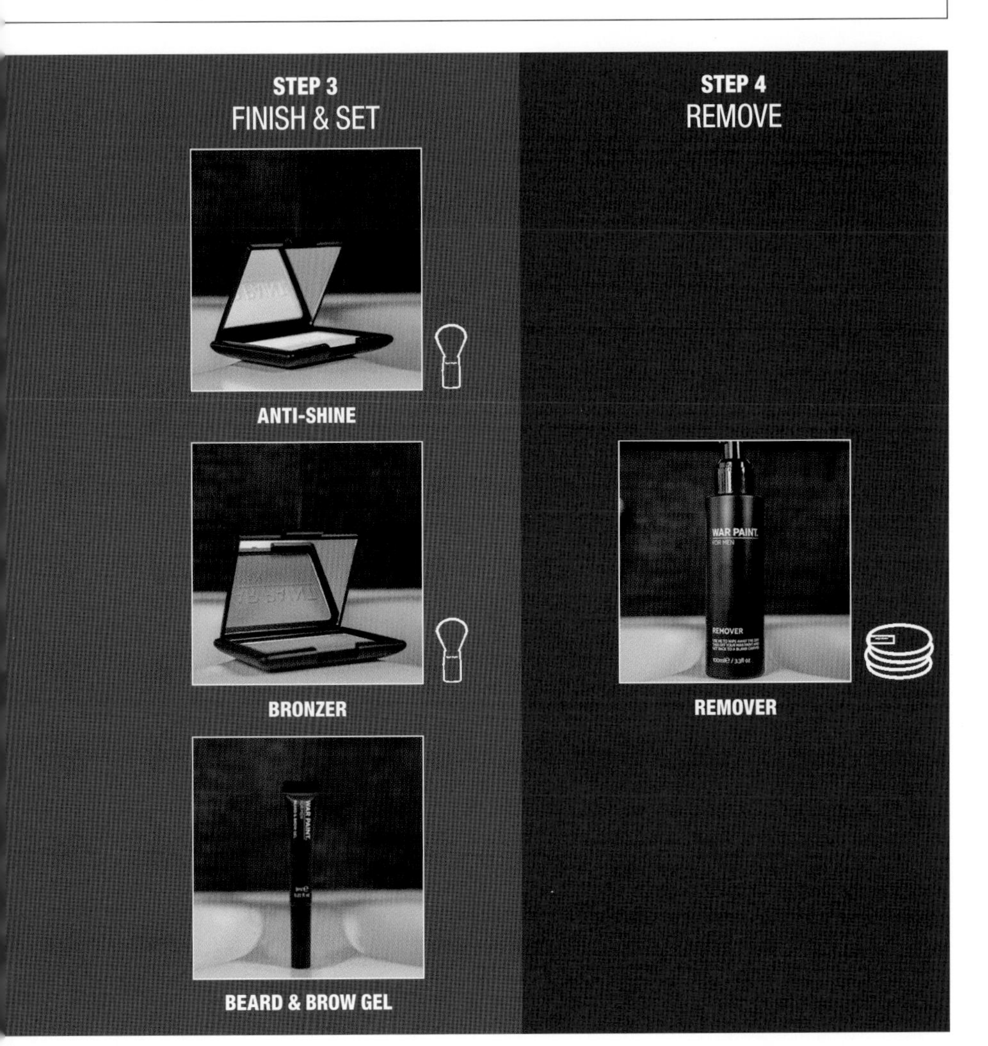

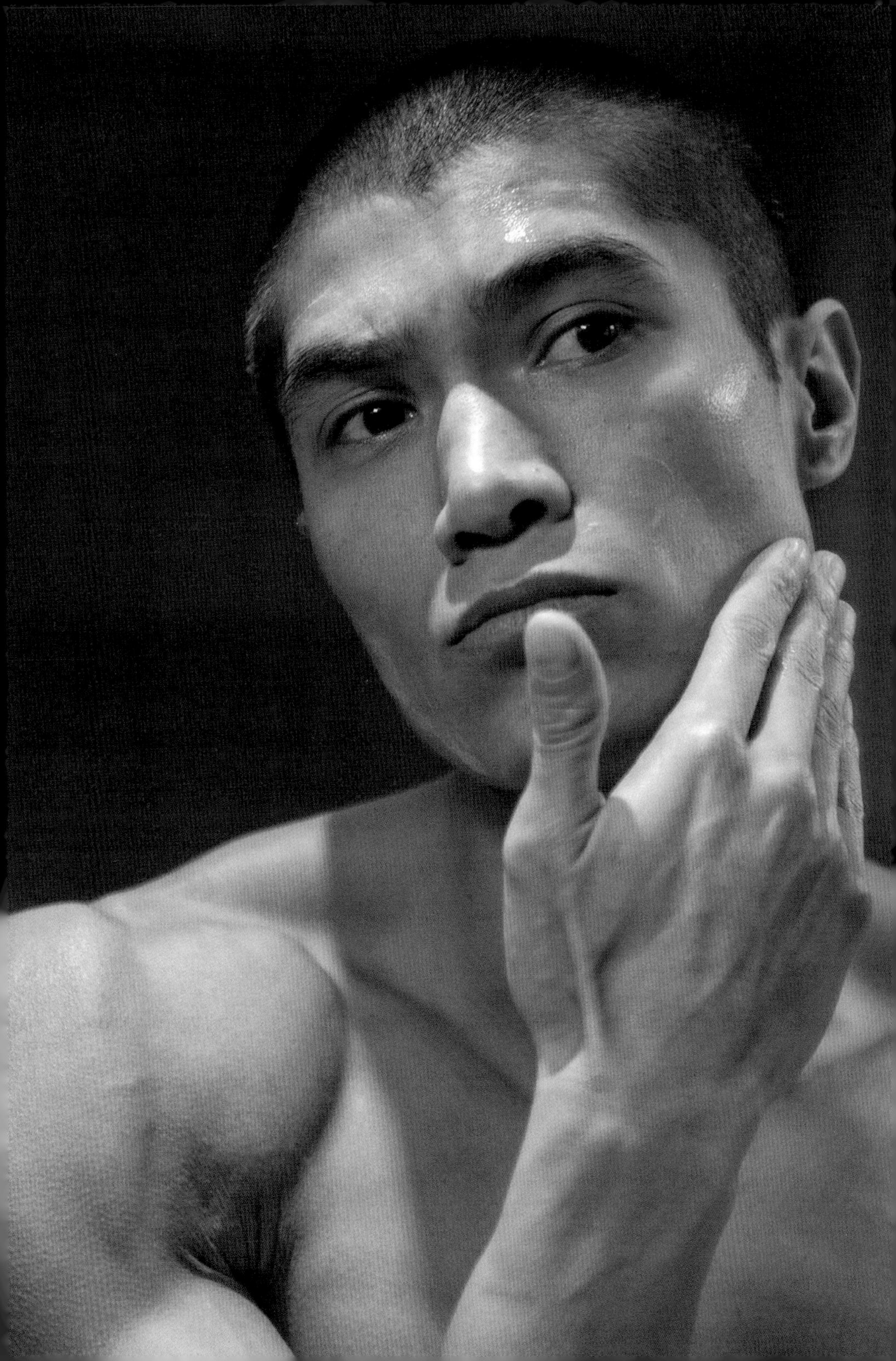

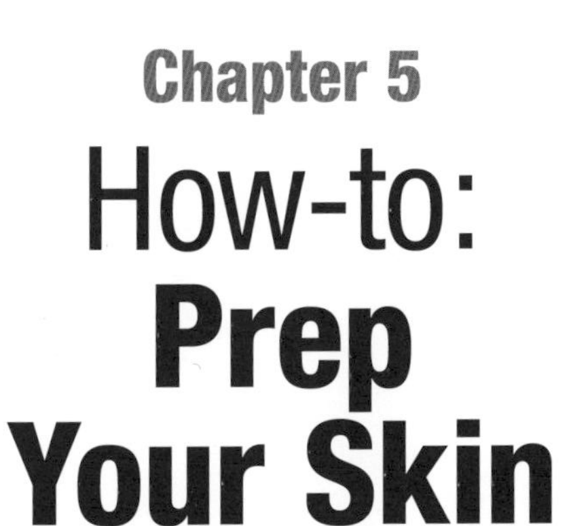

Chapter 5

How-to: **Prep Your Skin**

We're all about the makeup – it's what we do – but don't underestimate the power of skin prep when it comes to achieving the best finish for your face. In this section, we tackle the big four: exfoliators, moisturisers, SPFs and primers. You don't always *need* to use them daily, but it helps.

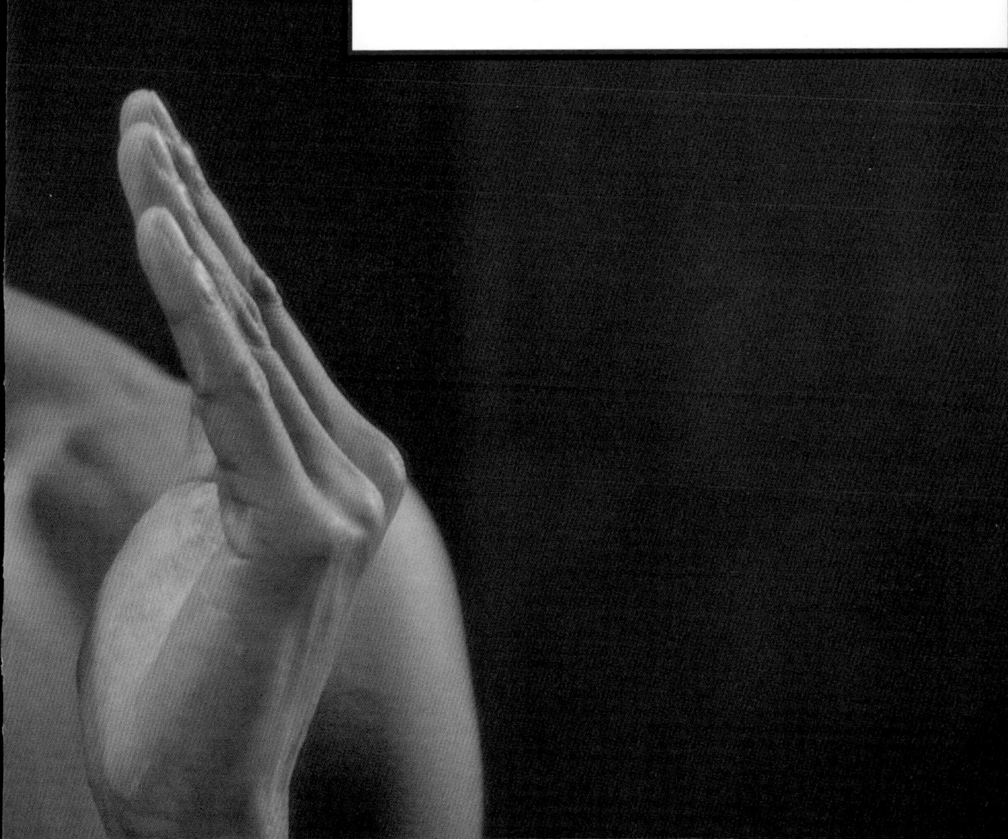

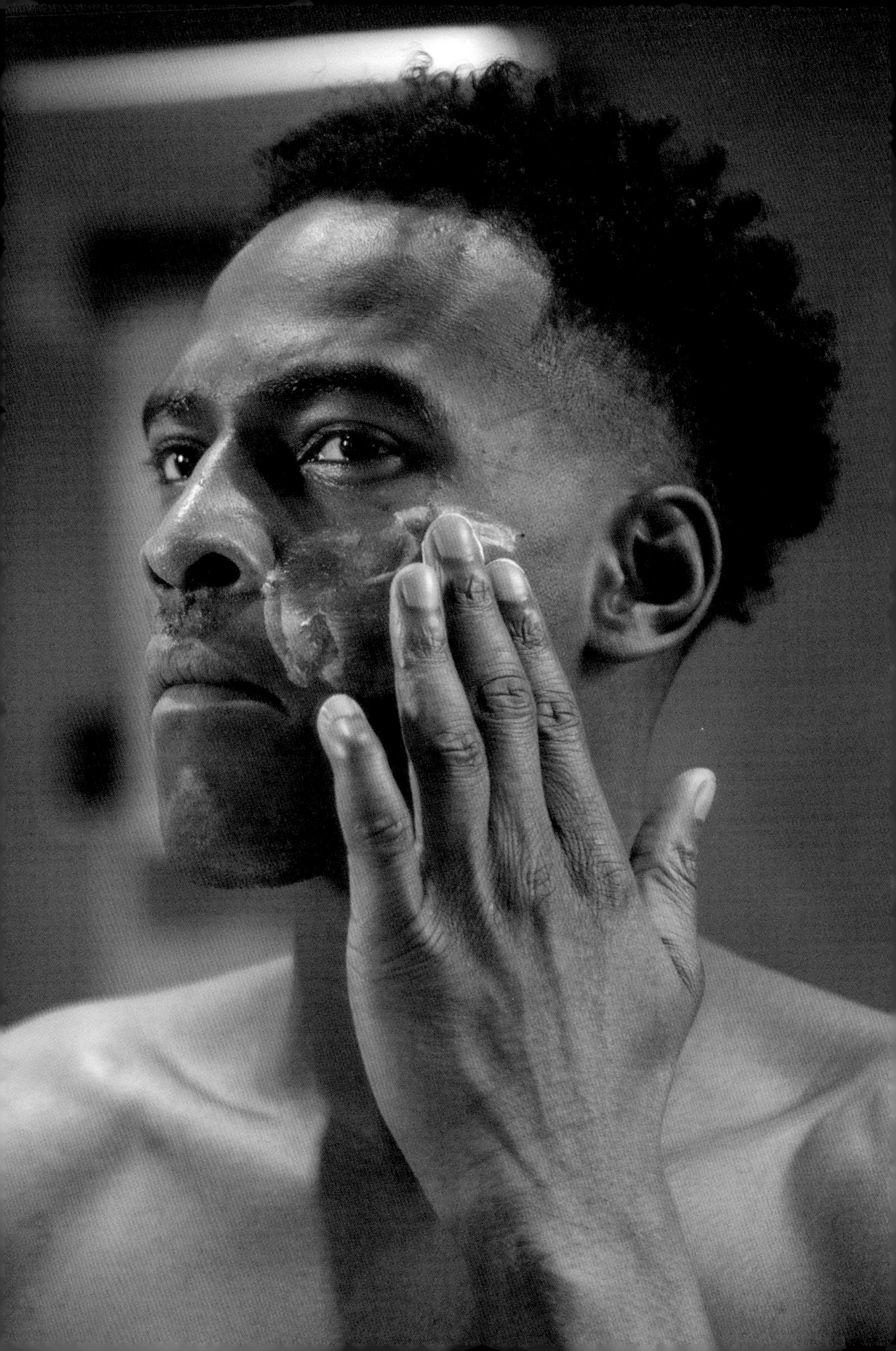

Exfoliate

Exfoliating is the unsung hero of skincare. It can tackle dryness, dullness and clogged pores – and results are pretty instant – so it's well worth having an exfoliating product on your bathroom shelf.

Why exfoliate?

Soap and water can only do so much. Think of exfoliation as a biweekly deep cleanse for your skin. Exfoliating buffs away dead surface cells, pore-clogging sebum and other debris that might have built up on your skin, so it can help prevent breakouts and ingrown hairs. A quick way of removing dead skin (it takes minutes), a good exfoliator can do everything from brightening your complexion to fading acne scars. Another bonus? It makes applying makeup easier, too, because you're working with a smoother canvas.

How often?

Although it's great in moderation, excessive exfoliation can aggravate your skin and cause redness, so try incorporating it into your regime no more than twice a week.

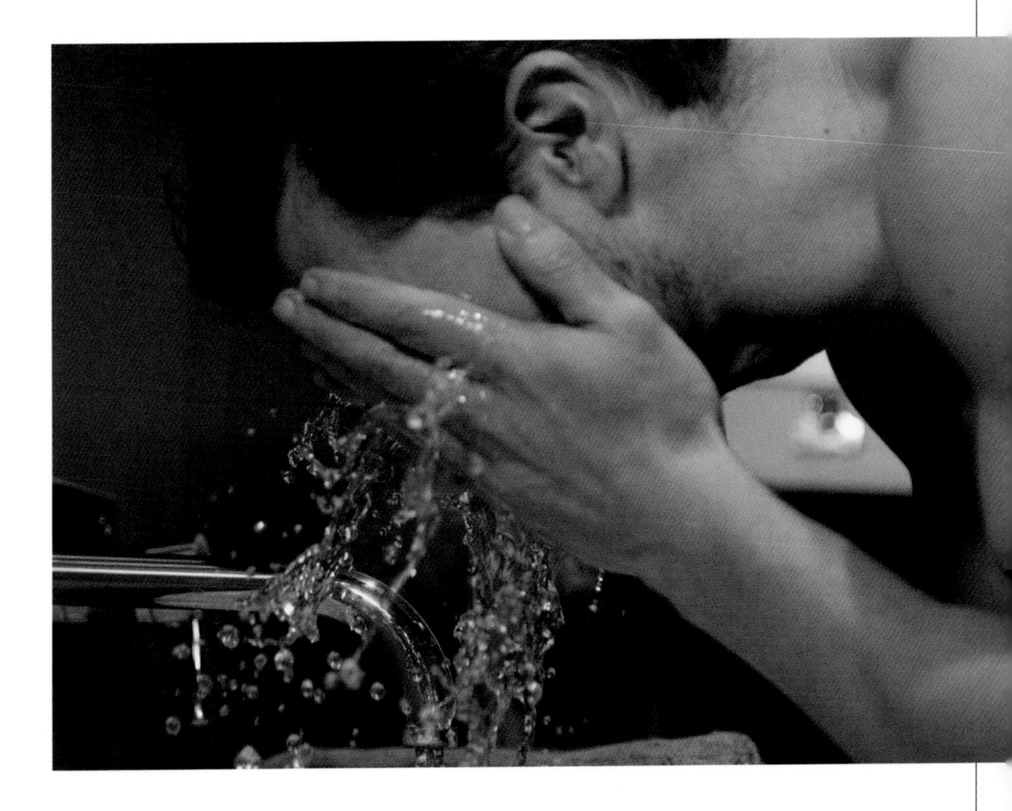

Types of exfoliators

There are two basic types of exfoliators, which can be equally effective, so it's all down to personal preference and what works best for your skin type. If in doubt, or you have sensitive skin, you're probably best off using a gentle exfoliator.

1. Physical exfoliator

Think of these as more like manual labour products that scrub your skin (but in a gentle way). Physical exfoliators use particles such as seeds, powders or rice granules to rub away the dead skin and leave it looking brighter and feeling smoother.

2. Chemical exfoliator

This sounds alarming, but it isn't. Usually, acids or enzymes help dissolve the bonds between cells and make it easier to buff away dead skin cells. The two most common chemicals used are alpha hydroxy acids (AHAs) and beta hydroxy acids (BHAs). An ingredient like glycolic acid can also help encourage new skin cell production so your skin instantly looks fresher. Chemical exfoliators can penetrate skin that bit deeper to improve the appearance of fine lines.

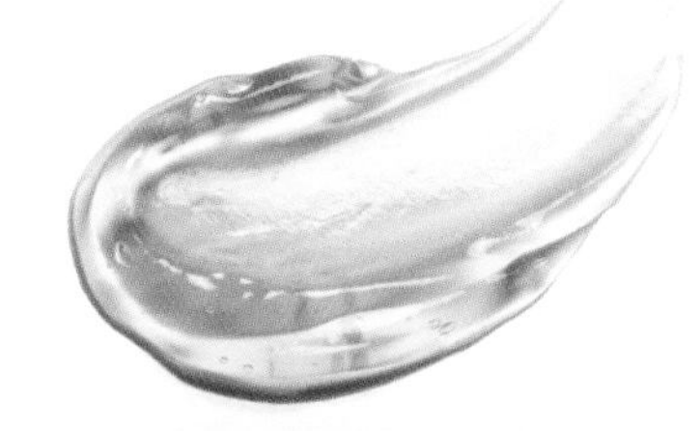

How to exfoliate

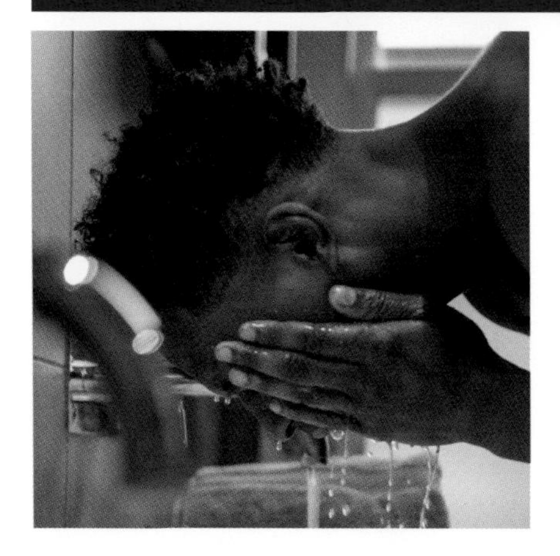

1 Use a face wash or daily facial cleanser to rinse away any dirt and excess oil and prepare your skin for exfoliation.

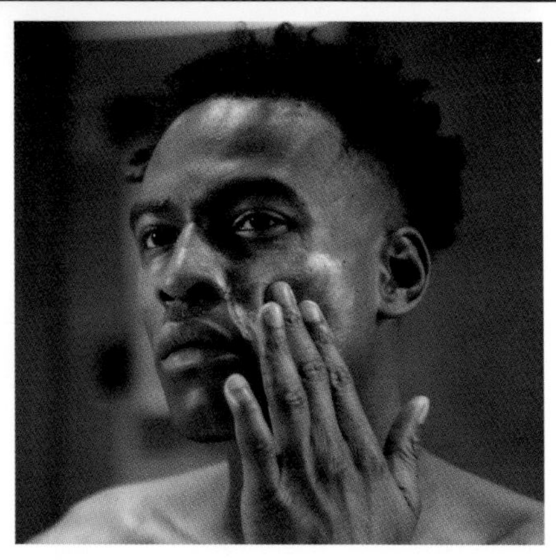

2 Most exfoliators work best on slightly damp skin (but always check the instructions). While your face is still damp, work in a coin-sized amount of product.

Tip

Beard or heavy stubble? Aim to extend the circular massage motion for another 5–10 seconds to allow the product to make full contact with your skin in that area.

Tip

If you have acne-prone skin, avoid abrasive physical exfoliators that contain harsh grains. Instead, use a chemical exfoliator, which will fight oil and acne at a deeper level in your skin.

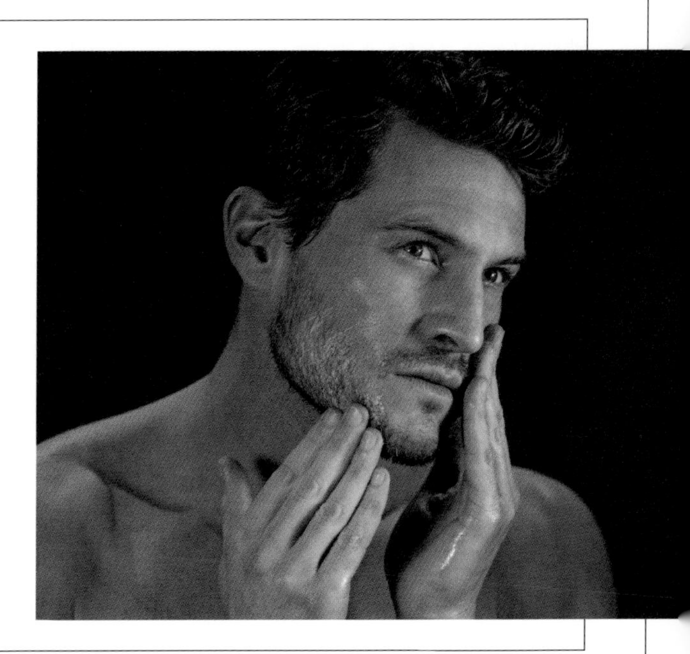

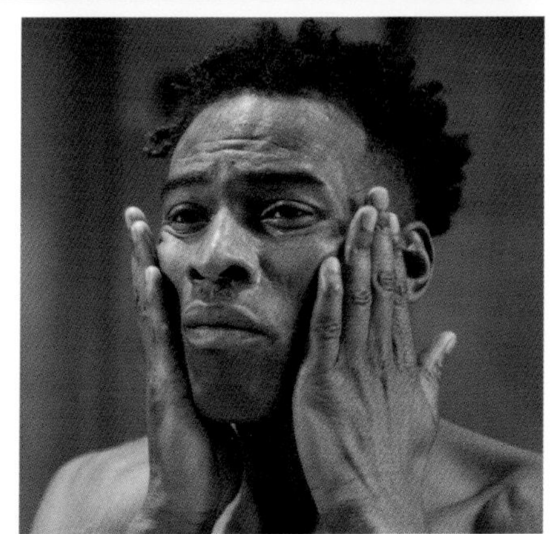

3 Gently massage it into your skin using a circular motion for 5–10 seconds. Rinse off thoroughly with lukewarm water and gently pat your face dry with a clean towel.

Do and don't

✓ Do use SPF afterwards. Exfoliating can make your skin more sensitive to sun exposure. If you're planning on spending a day in the sun, it's best to apply your exfoliator at night to give your skin time to recover.

✗ Don't exfoliate more than two or three times a week. Going overboard can result in redness and irritation so take it easy.

Moisturise

A moisturiser should be a core product in your skincare routine. Find a good one, and it will be your defence against not only the elements, but also the years. Use it twice daily and you'll wonder how your skin ever coped without it.

Why moisturise?

We're big fans of giving our skin the H_2O it needs. Some 64% of our skin is water, so the hydration you can get from a tub of moisturiser is basically like giving your skin a shot of water.

Let's be realistic, a moisturiser can't work Benjamin Button-style miracles, but start early and stay consistent and you could outsmart fine lines and wrinkles before they even start to appear. Invest in a moisturiser that works for your skin type (more of that on page 47) and it will not only help combat the early signs of ageing, but also keep extreme dryness or oiliness in check.

Today's high-tech, multitasking moisturisers do more than just the basic act of hydrating your skin, too. They provide protection from invisible environmental stressors, such as pollution, that age the skin – well worth considering if you live in the city.

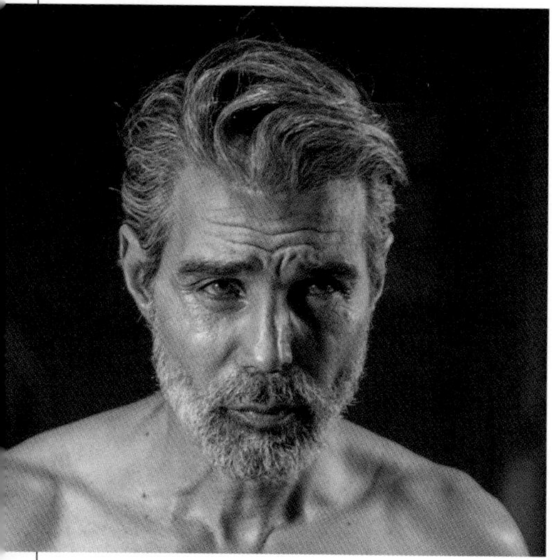

How often?

Getting into a regular routine is key when it comes to moisturiser. We know it's not easy to stick to the habit of moisturising as often as you clean your teeth, but the difference you'll notice in the elasticity and texture of your skin makes it worth doing twice daily. If you can tack on 90 seconds to your regime after you brush your teeth to give your skin some TLC, you're on to a winner.

A good daily routine would be to wash your face with a mild cleanser and follow it up with a moisturiser once in the morning and again at night. This simple but effective regime will keep your pores clean and your skin well hydrated.

If you want to go the extra mile and boost the potency of your moisturiser with a serum, check out our section on skincare extras on page 58.

Tip

Seasonal shifts mean your skin changes throughout the year so your moisturiser might need to follow suit. Try using a lightweight lotion in summer and switch to a thicker, richer formulation in winter to adapt to your skin's needs.

What's my skin type?

Is that generic special offer tube of moisturiser from the supermarket shelf not cutting it? Finding the moisturiser for your specific skin type is key so that it can deliver the benefits you need. Whether you want a mattifying lotion for oily skin or a super-hydrating formula to tackle dryness, a more targeted approach is where it's at when it comes to your moisturiser. Follow our simple breakdown to identify your skin type:

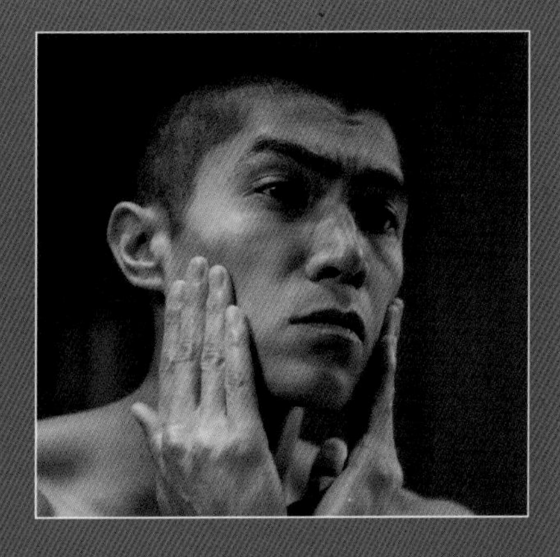

Dry skin

- Tight and flaky skin, with possible premature wrinkles
- Almost invisible pores
- Dull, rough complexion
- Rough and scaly texture
- Occasional red patches

YOU NEED: A moisturiser containing hyaluronic acid to give your skin a much-needed hydration boost.

Normal skin

- Generally, normal skin is described as neither oily nor dry
- Few imperfections
- Little or no sensitivity
- Barely visible pores
- Radiant complexion

YOU NEED: A good all-rounder moisturiser with hyaluronic acid for a hydration boost.

Oily skin

- Shiny or greasy-looking skin
- Enlarged pores
- Thicker-feeling complexion
- Blackheads, especially around the T-zone (see page 82)
- Pimples or blemishes

YOU NEED: An oil-free moisturiser in a light formulation to prevent pores from becoming clogged.

Combination skin

- Dry or normal in some areas and oily in others
- Pores that look larger than normal
- Blackheads
- Shiny skin, especially around the T-zone (see page 82)
- Dry skin in places

YOU NEED: A moisturiser that's specifically formulated to tackle combination skin. Application is key here: apply more product to the drier areas of your face, such as the cheeks, and go sparingly on the oilier parts of your face, to help balance out your skin.

Day vs night moisturiser

So you think you've found the holy grail of moisturiser, but does it work for day and night? It's a no-brainer to wear SPF in the day, but if your daytime moisturiser contains it, skin care professionals advise that you need a different moisturiser for night-time. Why? Because certain sun protection ingredients can clog up pores, especially in skin types that are prone to congestion and breakouts.

To spell it out in simple terms, SPF moisturisers have been engineered to be used during the day, while night creams have been designed to be used overnight when your skin is repairing itself as you sleep. Typically, night-time formulations are ultra-hydrating and contain specific active ingredients, such as peptides, to boost the skin regeneration process.

If a moisturiser double act – day and night – sounds excessive, go for a general all-rounder and apply your SPF separately.

Tip

Can you just borrow the moisturiser your missus uses? Your skin is likely to be about 23% thicker than hers and a completely different texture and type. If you're going to the effort of moisturising daily, use a type that works for *your* skin (and avoid the earache when she finds out you've been dipping into her designer cream).

How to apply moisturiser

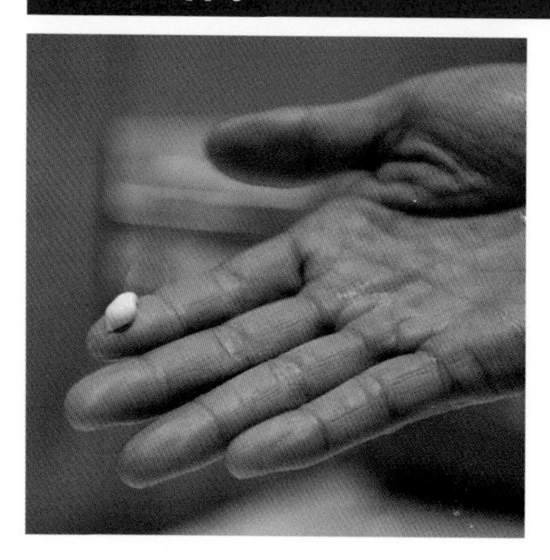

1 Squeeze a penny-sized amount of moisturiser on to your fingertips.

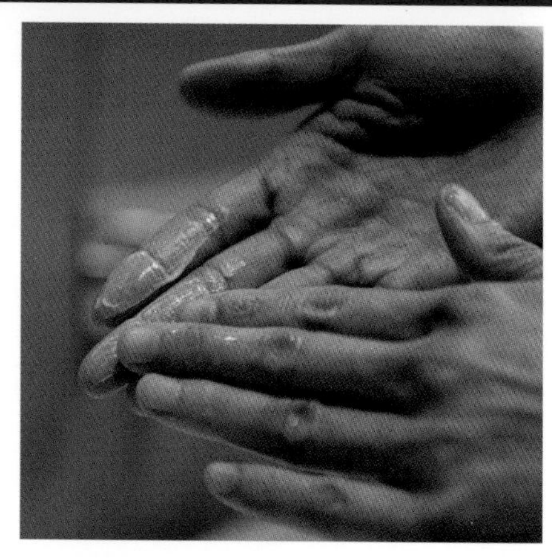

2 Rub your fingertips together to make it easy to distribute the product.

When to moisturise

Besides the obvious morning and night timeframes, moisturisers work hardest when they're applied to freshly cleaned skin. Doing this prevents your moisturiser from absorbing oil and impurities, which can cause breakouts. Aim to apply your moisturiser straight after cleansing when your face is towel-dried and still slightly damp.

No matter what your skin type, the skin on your face behaves differently in winter and often feels dry and tight – you can thank the constant switch between cold weather and central heating for that delight. So, if you feel like you're cracking up in the middle of the day and you've got some moisturiser to hand, go for a daytime top-up. It's no different to whipping out the hand cream to treat chapped hands.

Tip

Don't forget about the skin lurking underneath your beard. It can get pretty dry, especially if you use a beard trimmer regularly. Try using a beard oil to keep both the skin and beard hair hydrated.

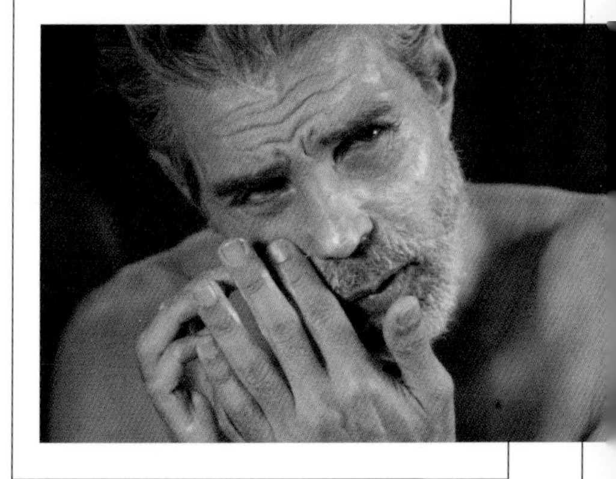

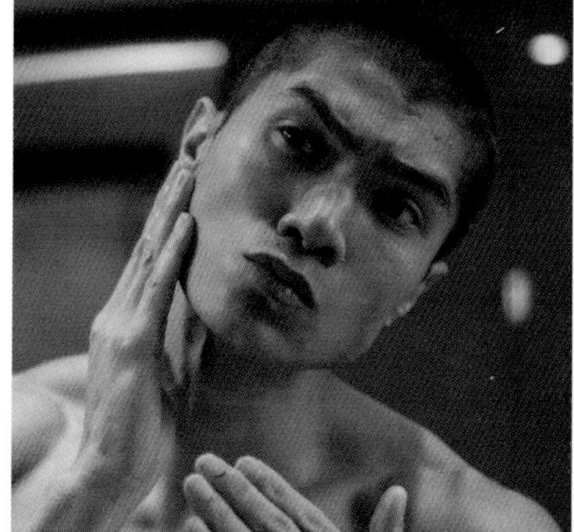

3 Apply the moisturiser all over and pay special attention to any areas that get particularly dry.

Do and don't

✓ Do always try to extend the moisturiser down to your neck where skin can get mega-dry from shaving.

✗ Don't apply moisturiser to your face when your skin is still soaking wet. Slightly damp skin immediately after cleansing is ideal because it helps to lock in the water.

SPF

You can't have a chapter on skin prep and not include SPF – it is non-negotiable in preventing sun-damaged skin. Try to get into the habit of applying suncare to your face every morning so you're all set for the day ahead.

Why use SPF?

There's a common misconception that you only need to wear SPF on vacation and during heatwaves to protect your skin. Think again. UV rays can penetrate your skin in any weather – on cloudy days, close to 80% of UV can still hit your face. Sun damage is no joke: apart from the onset of signs of premature ageing, such as wrinkles and sun spots, skin cancer is a life-threatening risk you shouldn't be taking.

To avoid ending up with skin like a weathered old boot, it's important to protect your face from sun exposure. Dermatologists advise wearing an SPF30 broad spectrum cream (which protects from UVA and UVB rays) on your face every. single. day. Yup, even when it's sweater weather.

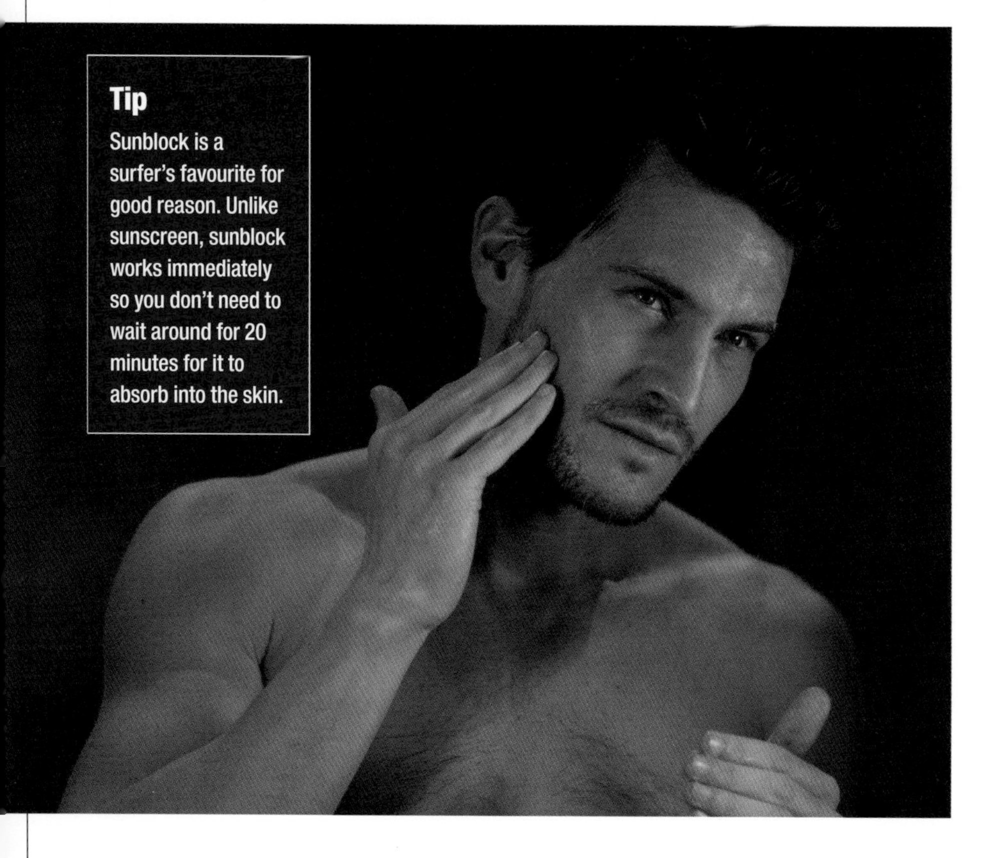

Tip

Sunblock is a surfer's favourite for good reason. Unlike sunscreen, sunblock works immediately so you don't need to wait around for 20 minutes for it to absorb into the skin.

How often?

Daily – unless you're planning on staying indoors for a hangover Netflix marathon. Even then, UV rays are so powerful they can penetrate windows (your car included). Play it safe and wear protection every day as part of your skincare routine.

How much and when?

The best way to apply facial suncare is to put on your regular moisturiser first, then apply a minimum SPF15 (though the higher the factor the better) every morning. Don't skimp on the amount – experts recommend about half a teaspoon for full-face coverage so make sure you slather it on generously. Aim to apply it about 20 minutes prior to sun exposure and reapply it every few hours on a particularly hot day.

What factor?

As a general rule of thumb, aim for a minimum of SPF15 for your daily face protection. But if you want to be extra diligent (and save your skin), dermatologists recommend SPF30 or above. If you have fair skin, you might want to consider using a higher SPF of 30–50.

Vacations require you to really up your suncare game in order to stay protected. Consider switching to SPF50 if you're jetting off to a hot country and your skin's likely to have prolonged sun exposure. You may be in holiday mode but remember to reapply suncare regularly, every two to three hours, to maintain the right level of protection – especially if you're in and out of the pool or tend to sweat a lot.

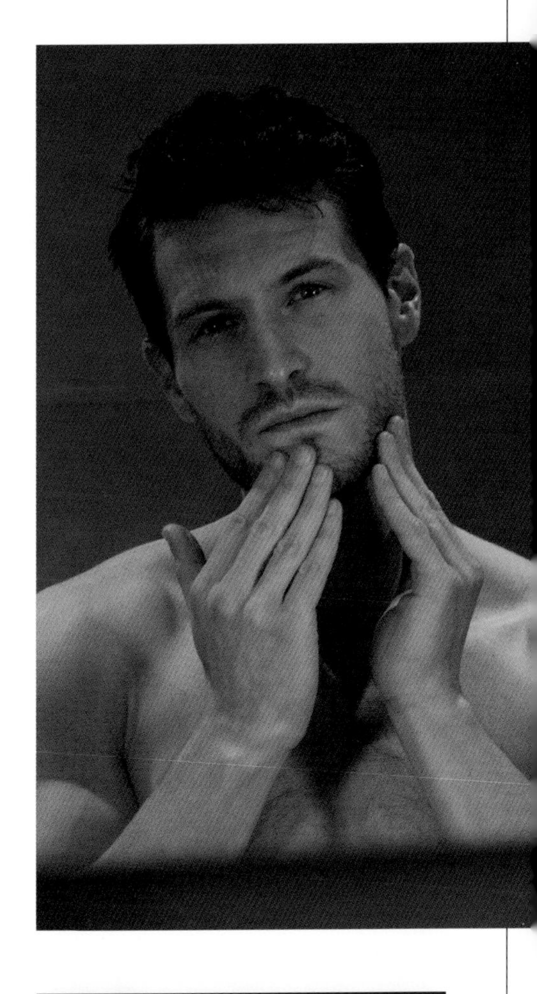

THE LOWDOWN:

Sun protection factor

SPF is the speedier way of saying 'sun protection factor'. The SPF number tells you what percentage of UVB rays are absorbed by the sunscreen. For example, SPF30 absorbs 97% of UVB rays – if you apply it with the correct thickness and frequency that is. SPF isn't an indicator of how long you can stay out in the sun.

Multitasking SPF products

We get that multitasking moisturisers with SPF are a great time-saver but, in reality, they're not as effective as a dedicated face SPF. Although it might say SPF15 in the small print, the amount that you put on your face is unlikely to be enough to get the full coverage that you need. Most SPF moisturisers aren't as hydrating as those without it, but wearing a day moisturiser with SPF is definitely better than applying no SPF at all.

Makeup, such as foundation containing SPF, is a similar story. You might just apply product where it's needed rather than the entirety of your face. In addition, mixing SPF with other ingredients dilutes the formula. We say, keep your SPF and makeup separate so you get the full benefit from your sunscreen.

> **Tip**
>
> **Always double-check the expiry date of your sunscreen before applying. Once opened, most SPFs will keep you protected for 6–12 months but always read the label. The safest bet is to ditch old product and replace it.**

Types of facial SPF

Cream

Similar to a moisturiser in texture, cream SPFs are the thickest in formulation so work well for hydrating normal to dry skin types. Because of their texture, it's worth noting that they can sometimes take a little more work to absorb into the skin.

How to apply SPF

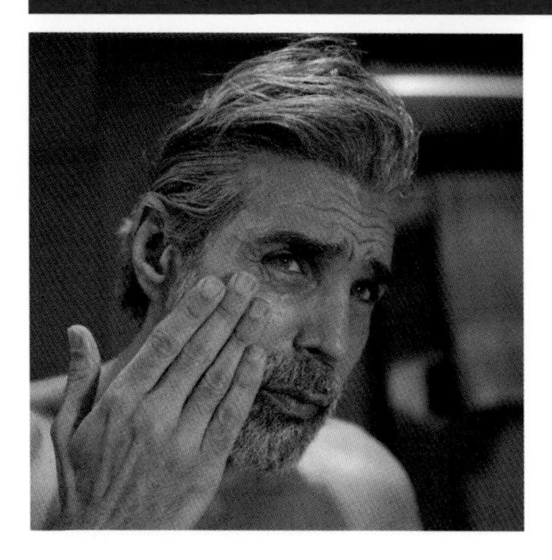

1 Apply your regular moisturiser all over your face.

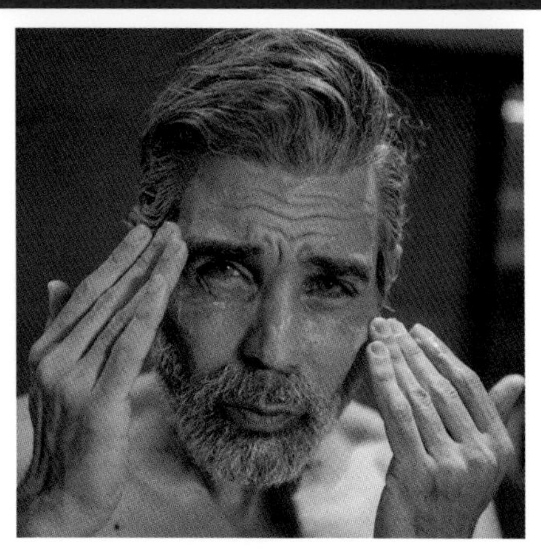

2 Once it's been absorbed, apply your SPF over the top at least 20 minutes prior to sun exposure.

Lotion

Somewhere between a gel and a cream, SPF lotions are a lightweight, hydrating option that absorb easily. If you have acne-prone or oily skin, go for an oil-free or non-comedogenic (minimum pore-clogging) option.

Gel

Gels have an almost water-like texture that glides on quickly. Cream sunscreens might leave behind white residue in facial hair (not a good look), so if you've got a beard or heavy stubble then a gel-based formula will be the easiest to massage in every morning.

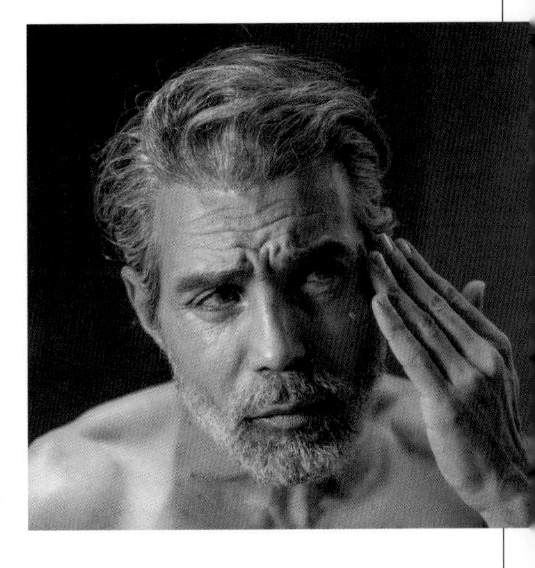

Stick

Handy for speedy, on-the-go applications, a stick SPF that you can throw in your pocket is best for targeted applications rather than the full face. Use a high SPF to slick over your nose, cheeks and tops of ears for extra protection on sun and ski trips.

3 Pay special attention to the tops of the ears and tip of your nose, where sunburn can strike.

Do and don't

✓ Do always be sure to apply sunscreen as the last step in your morning skincare routine – after moisturiser but before makeup.

✗ Don't mix your foundation or tinted moisturiser with suncare before application as it can disrupt the effectiveness of both products. Instead, apply your sunscreen before makeup.

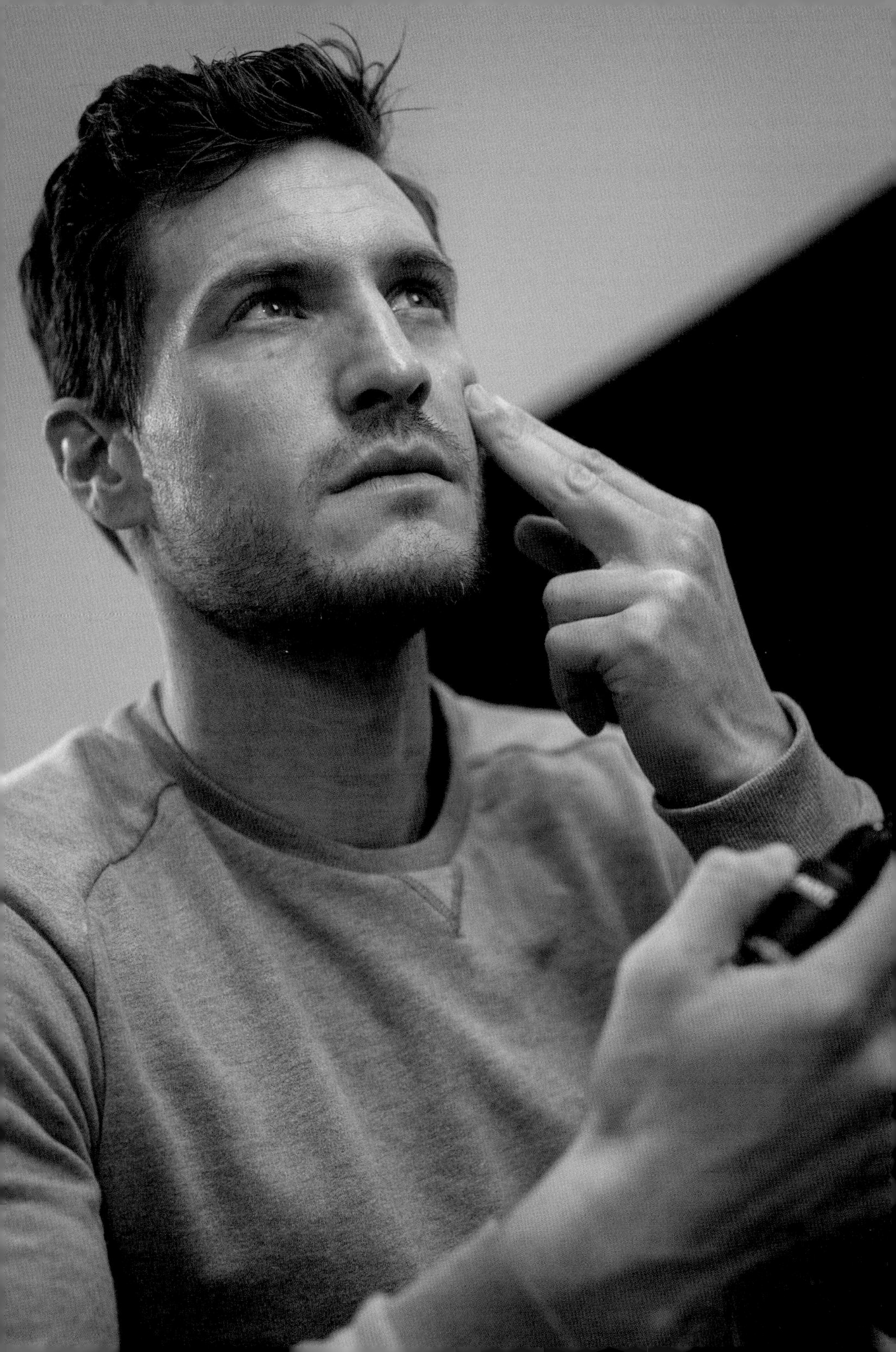

Primer

Primer is one of those cool hybrid products that's part skincare, part makeup. We're classing it as prep because it acts as the canvas for your makeup. It not only guarantees you a smooth, even base but also gives your finished look serious staying power.

What is primer?

Primer nearly always comes as a clear, gel-like liquid meaning it's invisible when it's on your skin. It's a product that professional makeup artists will always reach for first in their kit because it smooths, de-shines and helps hold your makeup, so is a real multitasking hero.

To get the smoothest base possible, apply it all over your face rather than to specific areas.

Tip

Donning a face mask out and about has become our 'new normal'. If you're wearing makeup, apply primer first to prevent any transfer on to your mask and ensure your base stays put when you take it off. Setting your base with translucent powder will also help your makeup go that extra mile.

Why prime?

If you're painting a door, you prime the surface first – and the same goes for your skin. Primer is your first port of call (after you've applied SPF, if you're using it): it will even out the surface of your skin and give your makeup a smooth, matte finish – ideal if you're prone to shiny skin.

Another benefit of prepping with a primer is that it gives your makeup endurance (we're talking morning commute to post-gym workout to beers with the lads) so it means you get way more out of your base, whether that's concealer, tinted moisturiser or foundation. Plus, it will give your skin that invisible boost to minimise your pores, smooth out blemishes and help control shine. A no-brainer.

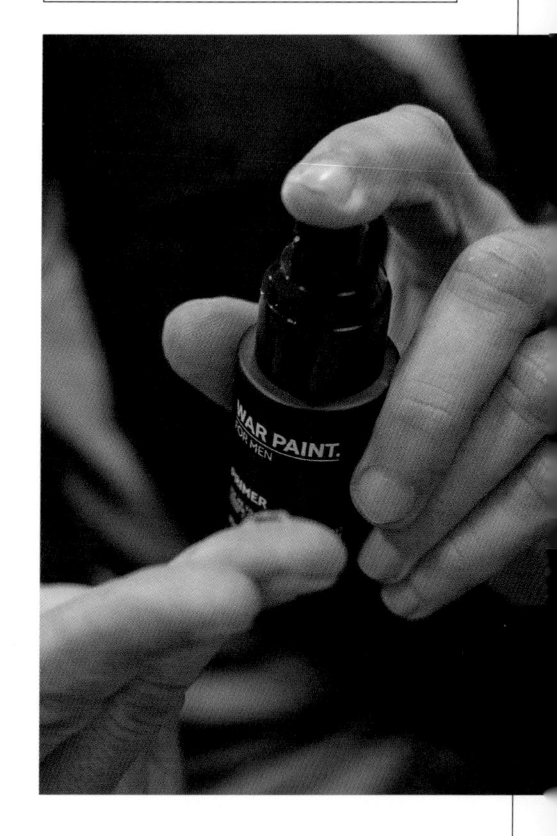

How often?

Unlike moisturiser or SPF, primer doesn't have to be a daily event. If you're happy with your skin's texture and how your foundation lasts, you may even decide that primer isn't for you. Or it might be that you only reach for it when you've got a full-on day and want to know your makeup will survive without top-ups.

For most guys, once they've tried using it and can see the benefits, it starts to feel like second nature to apply it before the chosen base. It really is a case of 'if you know, you know' (trust us).

When to use primer

There's no rulebook when it comes to makeup of course, but it may not surprise you to hear that primer comes first in the line-up – before any of your other makeup products.

Apply it after moisturising and using SPF and before applying your foundation, concealer or tinted moisturiser. Acting as a type of barrier between your skin and makeup, this will guarantee you a smooth base. Because of its gel-like texture, it's quick to apply and absorbs instantly, so there's no waiting around.

> **Tip**
>
> **Primers not only help even out your skin, but they also stop your foundation from slipping into fine lines and help smooth out wrinkles, so they act as a temporary anti-ager, too.**

How to apply primer

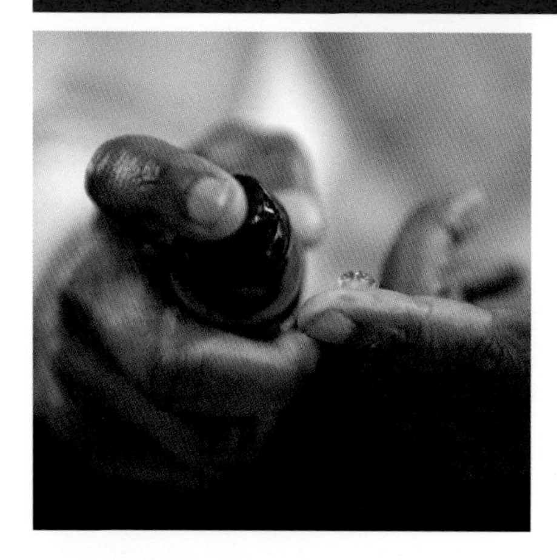

1 Apply one or two pumps of primer directly on to your skin with your fingertips.

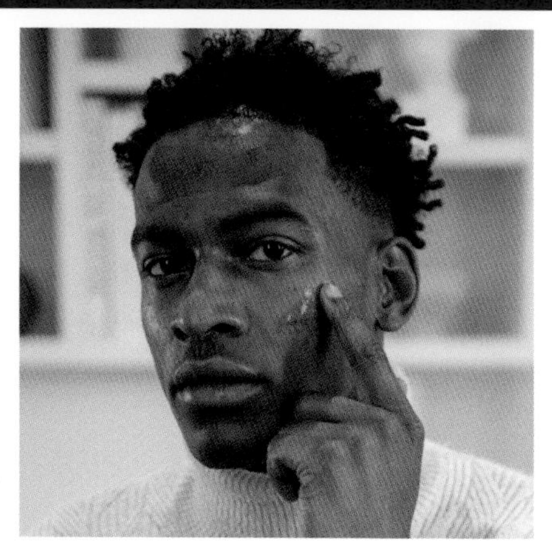

2 Smooth it over your face evenly, just like you would a moisturiser.

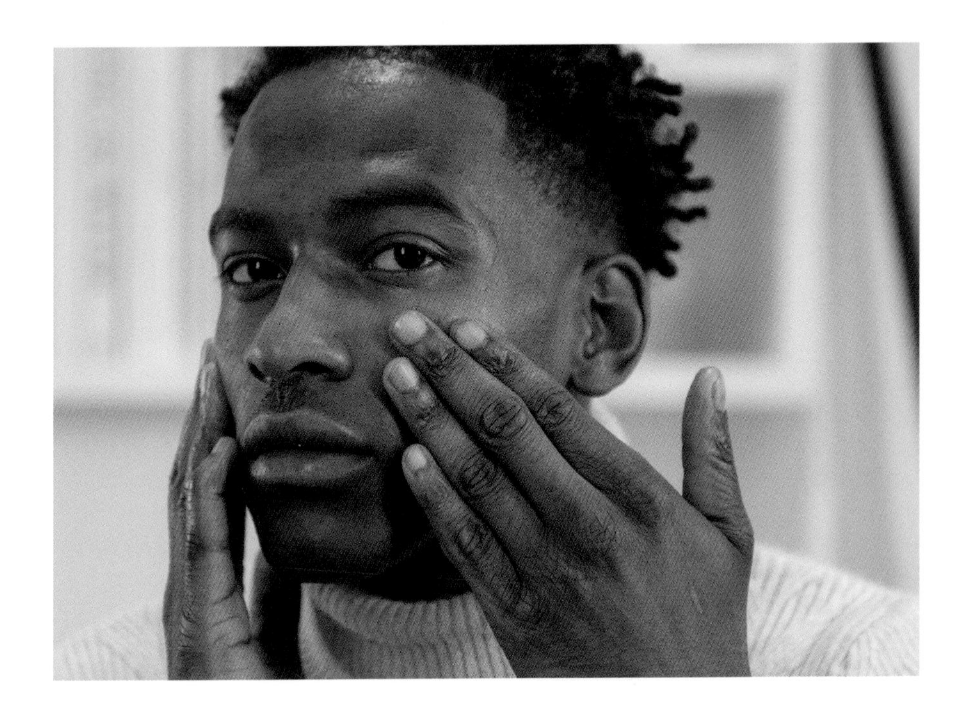

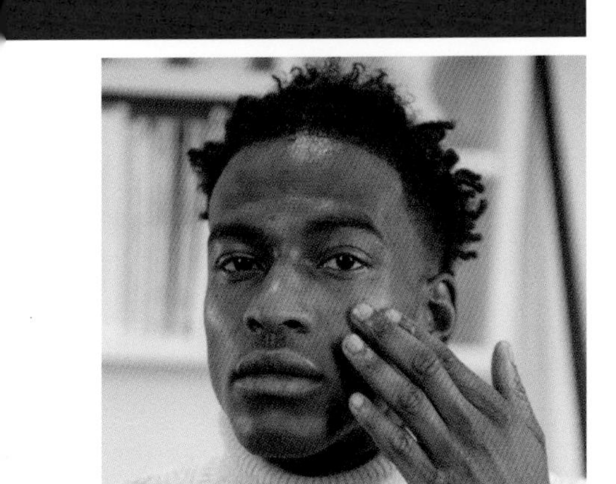

3 Wait a minute or two before applying your first makeup product.

Do and don't

✓ Don't apply too much primer. A little goes a long way so just one or two pumps should be enough to cover your whole face.

✗ Do always remember to wash your hands before applying primer to avoid the transfer of bacteria on to your skin.

Scan to watch the **'How to apply primer'** step-by-step video

Skincare extras

Just like makeup, skincare for men is booming right now. That's great news for increasing choice but also means it can be a minefield when it comes to navigating what should and shouldn't make the cut in your bathroom cabinet. If you want to go beyond the core products, these are the extras to consider adding to your shelf. Welcome to the big league.

Serum

More potent than your average moisturiser, serums differ because they deliver product directly into your skin instead of remaining on the surface. It might sound a little sinister but that means the product is targeting the dermis beneath the top layer of skin to deliver active ingredients and also tackle any specific issues that your skin might be facing, such as ageing or outbreaks.

Brand new to serums? Pick up a good all-rounder that contains skin-building ingredients such as hyaluronic acid and vitamin C. Use a serum after cleansing and before your moisturiser for the most effective results.

Masks

From sheet masks for men to overnight sleep-ins, there are hundreds of different kinds of masks out there for multiple skin concerns. One thing they all have in common is that they're designed to supplement your core skincare routine – they're not a daily addition alongside your SPF or moisturiser. Think once or twice a week to tackle a key concern.

Perfect for a fast fix, face masks are turbocharged with active ingredients to help you tackle everything from dry patches to blemishes. If in doubt, let the key ingredient guide you. For example, activated charcoal is known to help detoxify and remove impurities from your pores.

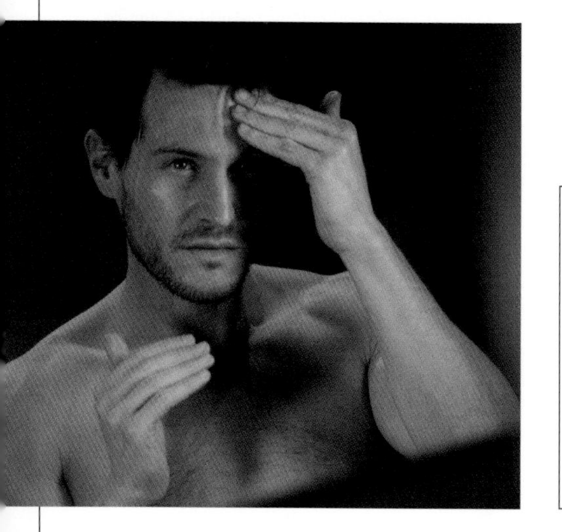

Tip

Using multiple skincare products? We salute your dedication. The order in which you apply them counts. Aim for the general rule of cleanse, tone, serum, moisturise, SPF, then eye cream. To make it easier to remember, the thinnest products always go first.

Preventing 'maskne'

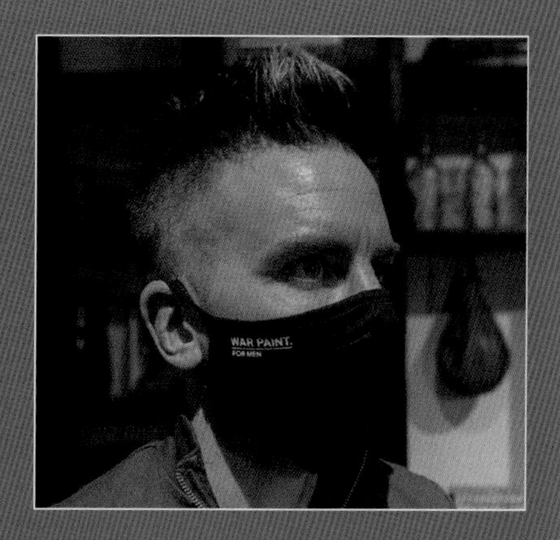

Before 2020, nobody had heard of the word 'maskne'. But what is it? It's all down to face coverings, which have become the unexpected must-have (and sometimes mandatory) accessory of the start of the decade. These come with a side effect: 'maskne', which is Covid-19 lingo for breakouts on your chin, jawline and nose caused by wearing face masks.

These happen thanks to the constant rubbing of the masks against our faces and by the moist environment going on underneath the masks, which creates a breeding ground for bacteria and dirt that can clog up our pores and cause breakouts. Here's how to prevent mask-induced acne.

- Always wash your hands thoroughly before donning your mask – it will help prevent the transfer of bacteria to your face.
- Choose your mask fabric wisely. A 100% cotton or silk mask is a better option for acne-prone or sensitive skin. Synthetics such as polyester and nylon are less breathable so there's a bigger risk of facial irritation.
- Aim to wash your reusable cloth mask after each use. If you're wearing it all day, change your face mask as soon as it gets damp or after a few hours of continued use.
- Avoid heavy-coverage makeup if you're going to be wearing a mask for long periods of time. If you have clean hands, you can always opt for the on-the-go approach and apply your base or concealer once you've stashed your mask away.
- If your maskne feels out of control and goes beyond a few angry spots, it might be time to call a dermatologist for advice on suitable treatments for your skin.

Eye cream

This is definitely an optional (and sometimes pricey) extra, but using a small amount of eye cream can help fix a whole host of concerns, from puffy under-eye bags to early signs of ageing. You might have noticed that the area around your eyes is thinner and the skin more fragile than it is on the rest of your face, so it's one of the first places where you can expect to see fine lines and deeper wrinkles, such as crow's feet, to appear.

If anti-ageing isn't a concern yet (lucky you), go for an all-purpose cream that can be worn to pep up your eye area both morning and night. Most eye treatments for men are engineered to invigorate tired eyes, de-puff bags and brighten up those dark circles so you can face the day looking fresher. If shine's a concern, look for an eye cream with a matte finish.

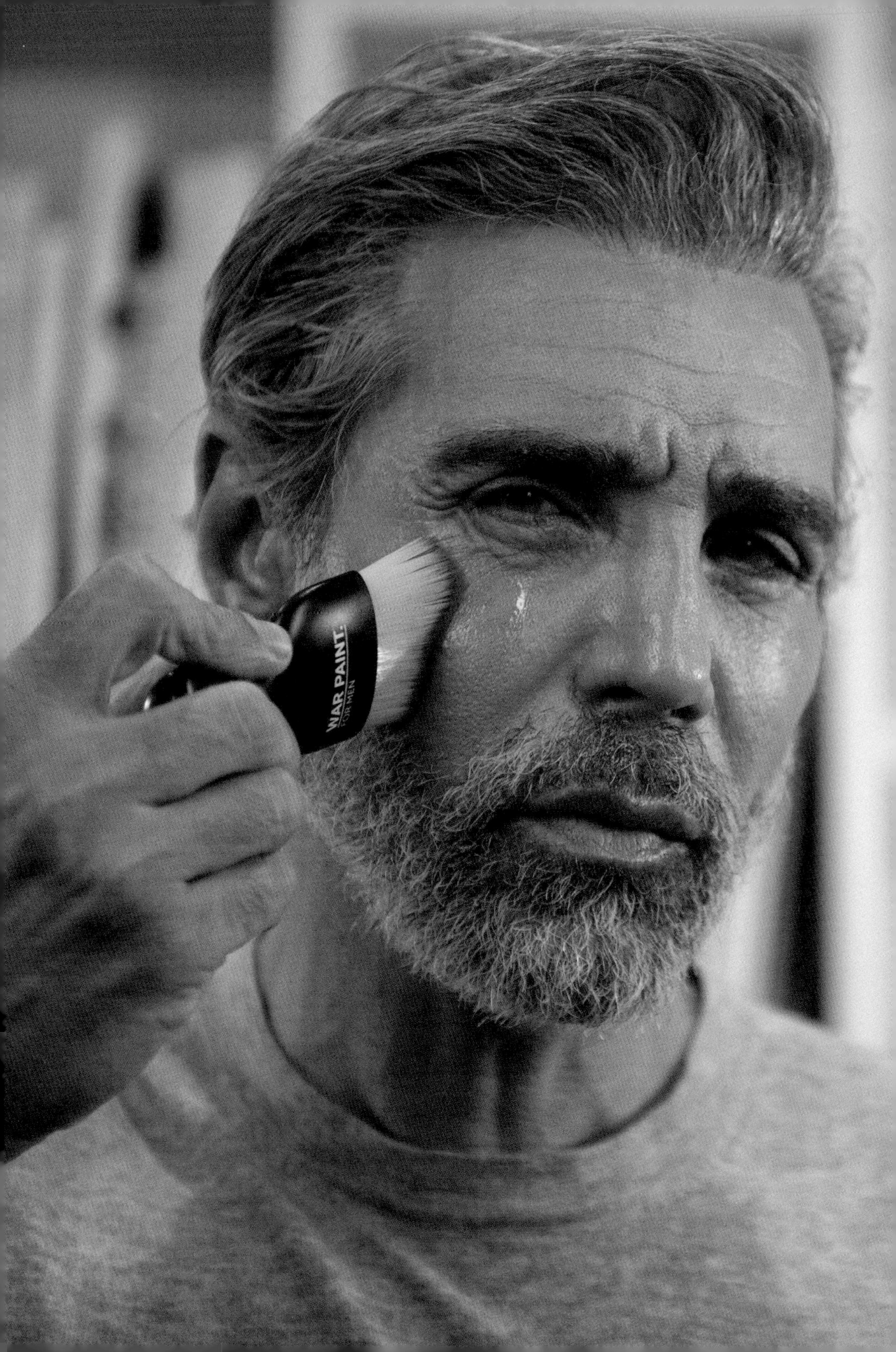
WAR PAINT.
FOR MEN

Chapter 6
How-to: **Even Out Your Skin Tone**

Evening out your skin tone might be subtle (we're all for the no-makeup makeup look) but, ultimately, it's the main reason men want to use makeup: so their skin looks fresher, smoother, blemish-free and maybe even a few years younger. Whatever the motivation, the result looks like your skin, but better.

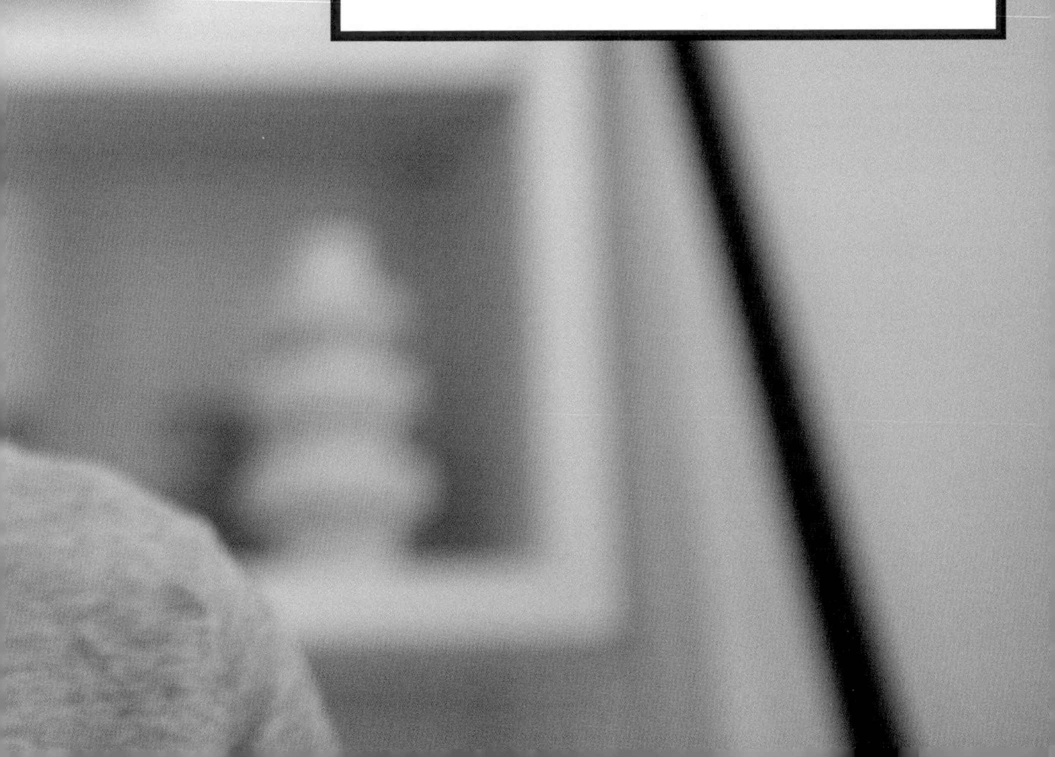

Concealer

Think of concealer as the jack of all trades in your kit bag. It's probably (read: definitely) the most versatile makeup product out there for us guys. You can either use it for targeted applications or apply it wherever you feel it's needed on your face to cover any areas of redness or imperfections.

What is concealer?

Like most men's makeup, it's not rocket science. As the name suggests, a concealer is a skin-toned cream or liquid that conceals just about every imperfection you can think of.

Why conceal?

Small but mighty, concealer is the shortcut solution to getting great skin (or at least looking like you have great skin). A good concealer can mask just about any unwanted mark on your skin, from hiding dark under-eye circles, to evening out skin tone, to making a spot disappear, pronto.

If you look in the mirror and pinpoint/swear profusely at something that's bothering you then a concealer is your instant quick-fix solution. Used correctly (which is where we come in), it will blend the imperfection into the surrounding skin tone so you can get on with your day feeling confident instead of self-conscious.

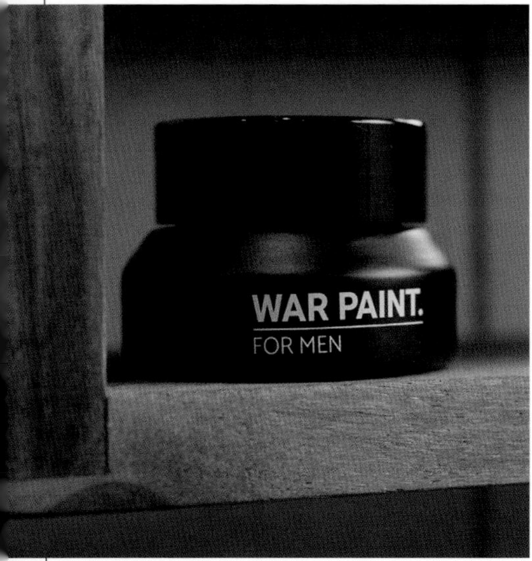

When to use concealer

Some guys use concealer every day without fail to even out their skin, others just pick theirs up for SOS when they have a specific imperfection they want to cover up, such as a post-heavy-night spot. Seriously, it happens to us all. Concealer can be a lifesaver if you want to blank out a blemish or an acne breakout and pretend it's not happening.

Unlike primer, which you always call on first, there's no set rule for when you apply concealer. You can use it before a foundation or tinted moisturiser, afterwards, or on its own. Powerful enough to go solo, a concealer doesn't have to be used in conjunction with a ton of other makeup products.

WAR PAINT.
FOR MEN

Tip

Layering up your concealer is a good tactic to know about. If you've used a tinted moisturiser or foundation and you can still see redness, dark circles or a spot, reapply your concealer on top of your base in the areas it's needed.

Find your concealer shade

Besides creating a two-tone face and neck, using the wrong-colour concealer is up there as one of the worst makeup offences you can commit. That all sounds worrying, but don't panic, we've got your back.

Some makeup professionals will argue that you can be top of your concealer game with two different shades: one that's one to two shades lighter than your natural skin tone to camouflage and brighten under-eye bags, and a second that's a close match to your skin tone for blemishes. Our take? We say go for one all-rounder that's closest to your skin colour, especially if you're just starting out with makeup.

How do you know if you've got the right shade? Pick a colour that's as similar to your current skin tone as possible, otherwise you'll just be drawing attention to the area. You know a concealer is the right shade for you because it will blend seamlessly into your skin tone with very little effort. Test out the colour on the area just below your ear around your jawline.

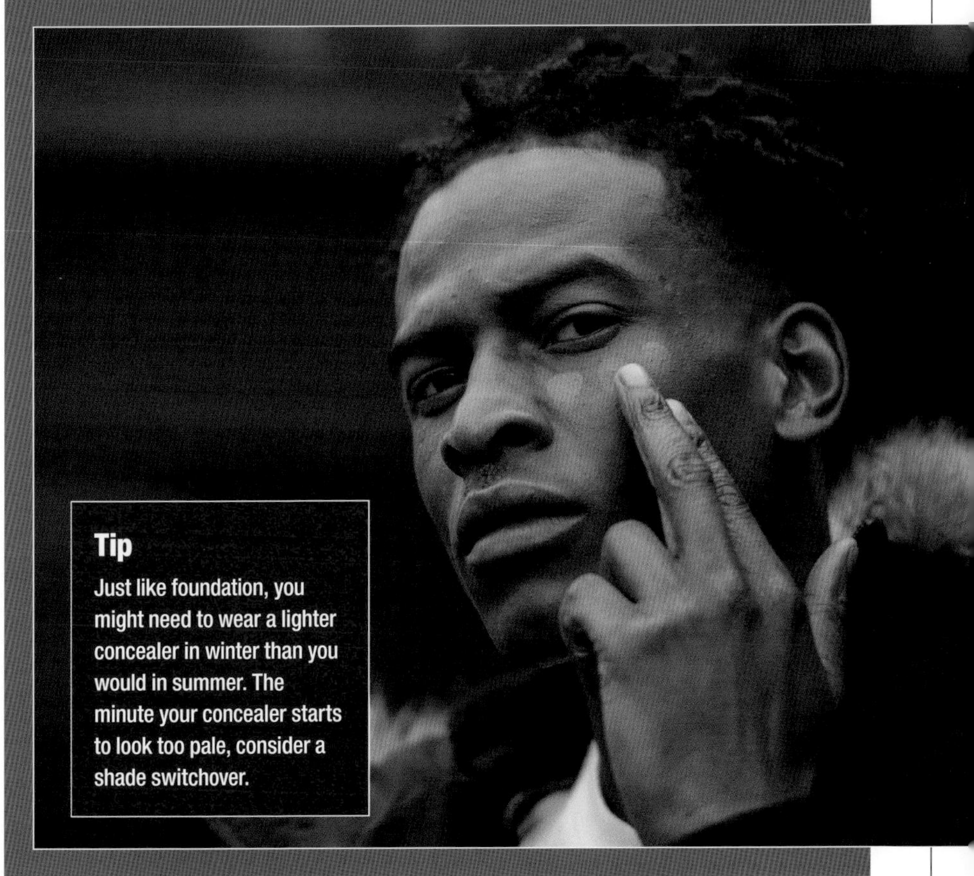

Tip

Just like foundation, you might need to wear a lighter concealer in winter than you would in summer. The minute your concealer starts to look too pale, consider a shade switchover.

How to apply concealer: Using your fingertip

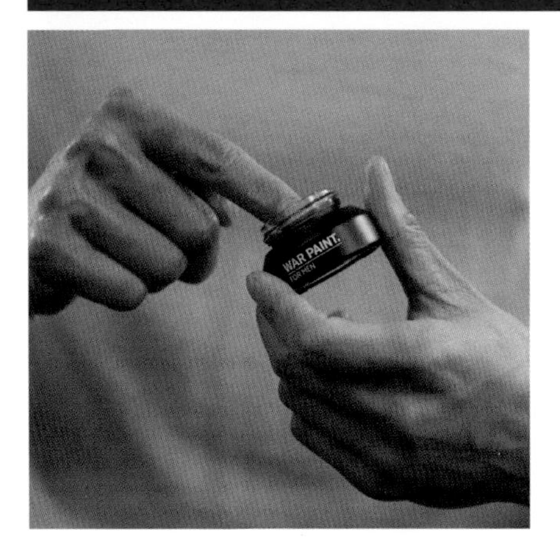

1 Use a clean fingertip to dot concealer lightly under the eyes.

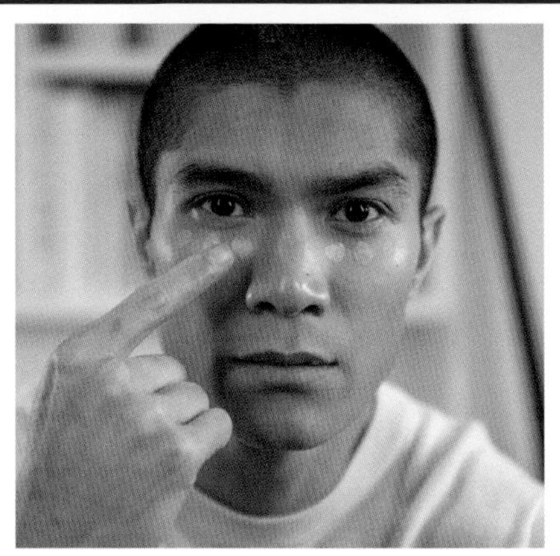

2 Once applied, use the same fingertip to dab and blend it into your skin.

How to apply concealer: Using a sponge

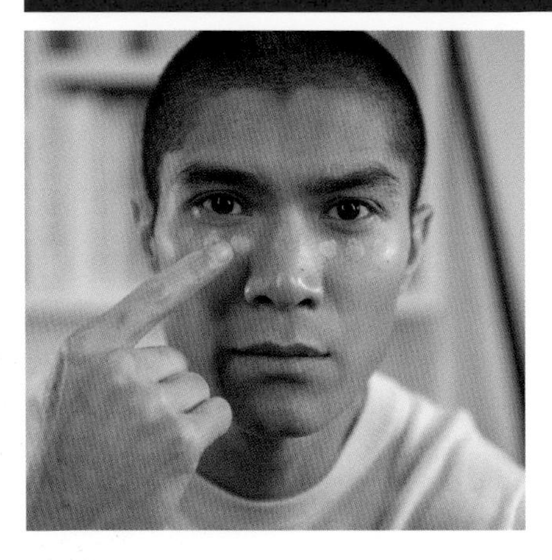

1 Dot concealer lightly under the eyes or on problem areas.

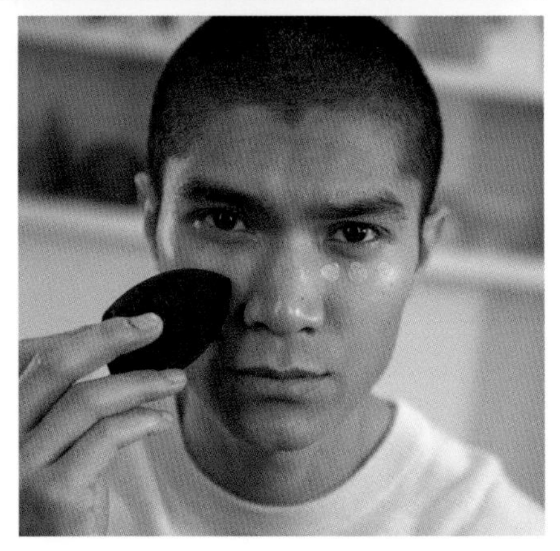

2 With a damp sponge, blend in the product across the face using a dabbing motion.

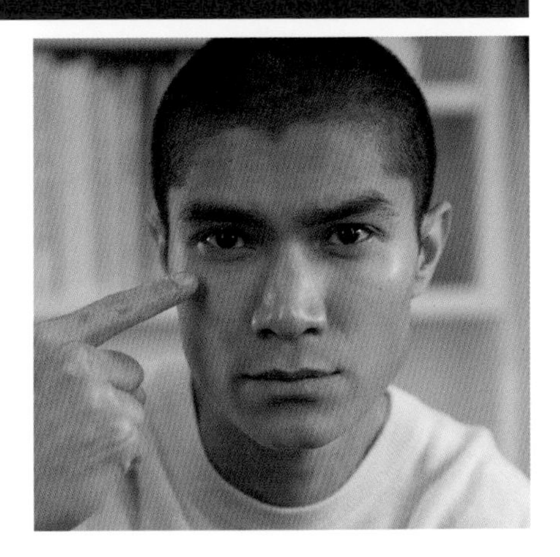

3 Smooth under your eye gently with your fingertip to ensure the concealer is fully blended and not sitting in any creases.

Do and don't

✓ Do get the shade right for your skin tone. Using a single layer of concealer that is very different from your natural skin tone can leave your skin looking worse rather than better.

✗ Don't rub your concealer in. When it comes to blending concealer, always dab. Rubbing can remove any base product you've already applied underneath.

Scan to watch the **'How to apply concealer'** step-by-step video

Say goodbye to dark circles

Heavy night? This is what concealer can do to eradicate your eye bags and dark circles – in seconds. Conceal, blend, done.

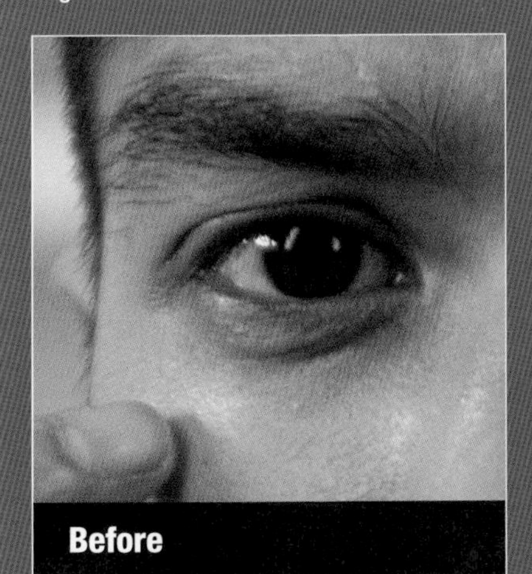

Before

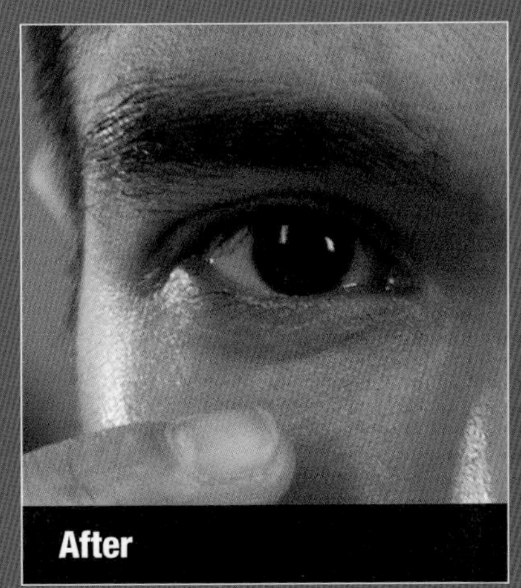

After

Hangover SOS

You can run (probably slower than usual), but you can't hide from a killer hangover. But makeup – namely concealer – is your get-out-of-jail-free card if you've got a 9am Zoom call looming with your boss and want to hide the evidence of an all-nighter.

Here are our tips for looking like you've had eight hours' solid sleep. Bacon sarnie, optional.

- First thing first: rehydrate your skin inside and out. Water helps to give your skin that healthy, hydrated look so neck a couple of glasses of H_2O.
- Hydrate the surface of parched skin by washing it with a good cleanser (cold water can help refresh) followed by moisturiser to wake up your face.
- If your skin's got that telltale hangover blotchiness or redness, reach for a tinted moisturiser to even everything out. Pop some on your hand and apply exactly like you would a moisturiser.
- Concealer is the heavy-night hero that will disguise under-eye bags and/or dark circles in seconds and make your eyes look fresher. Use a clean fingertip or a brush or sponge to dot concealer lightly under the eyes and blend it in.
- A heavy night of booze (and 2am takeaway) can sometimes result in redness around the nose and cheeks. Use your concealer to camouflage any red zones, building up the coverage lightly with your fingertip, brush or sponge.

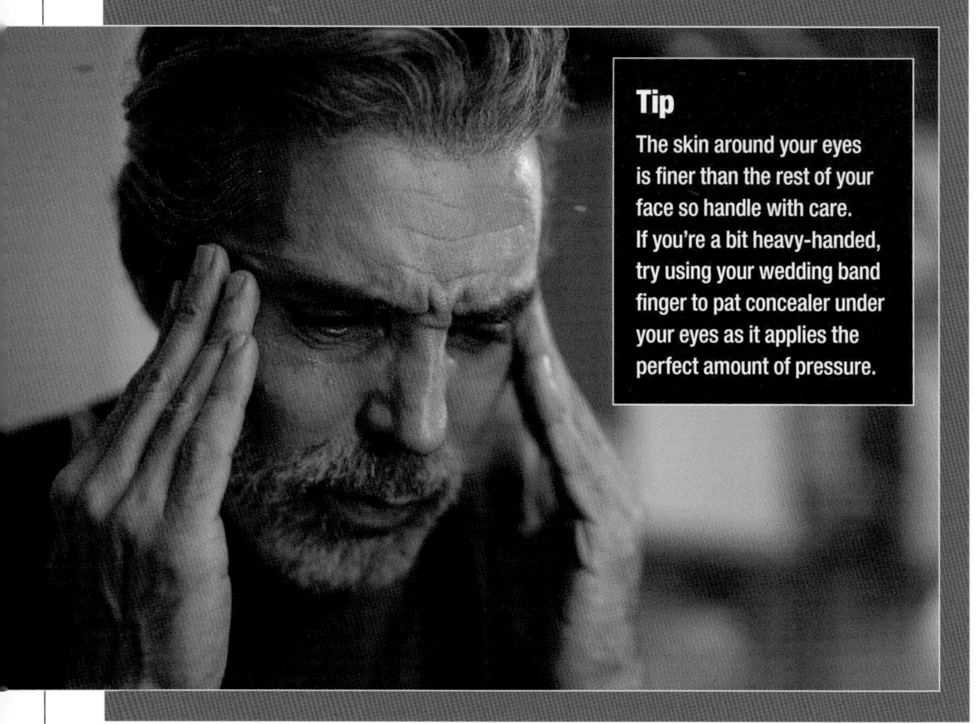

Tip

The skin around your eyes is finer than the rest of your face so handle with care. If you're a bit heavy-handed, try using your wedding band finger to pat concealer under your eyes as it applies the perfect amount of pressure.

Concealing a bad breakout

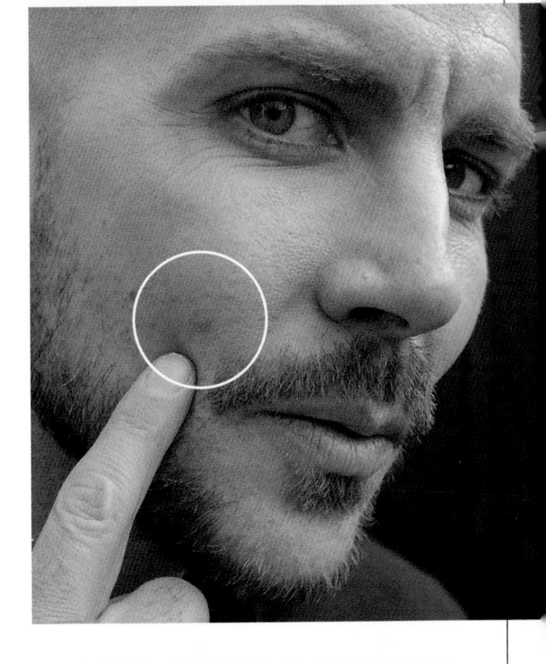

We're a makeup manual so we're not going to delve into treating acne and breakouts (a good dermatologist can do that), but we are pros at covering spots with makeup. Cue the concealer stick.

Don't panic if that big spot feels like it's taking over your face. These are our three hacks for covering up blackheads, blemishes and acne breakouts in seconds.

1 When you conceal a blemish, you don't want it to break out more. Always make sure you're using a clean fingertip, brush or sponge to apply your concealer.

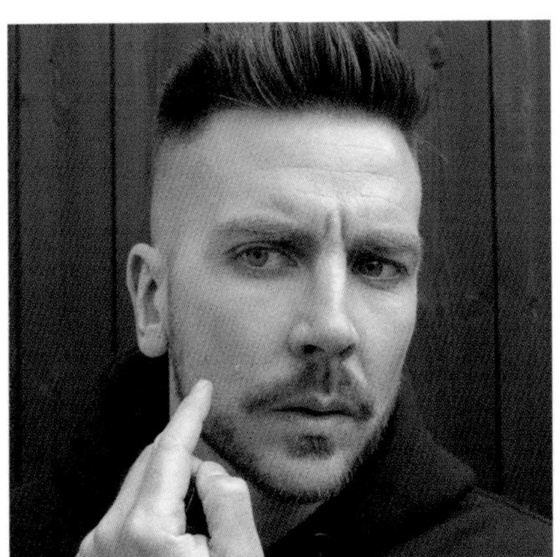

2 Put just enough concealer on the spot to cover up any redness. Then to conceal your concealer, add a thin layer of foundation (the same colour as your natural skin tone), to make the blemish less noticeable.

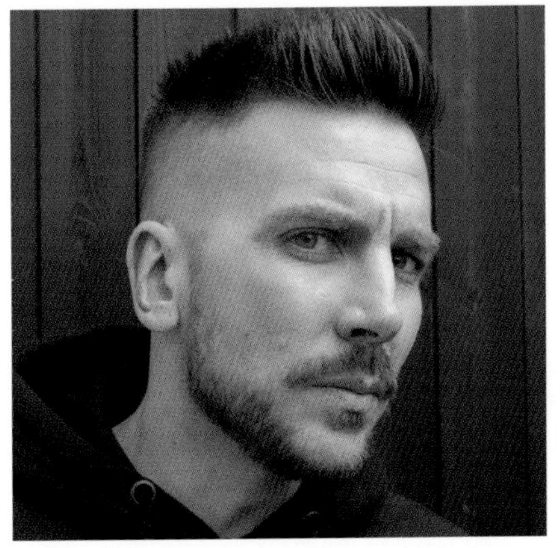

3 If a big spot is still showing through (it can happen), tackle it after applying the rest of your makeup. Add just a dot of concealer over it as the last step in your makeup routine.

Tinted moisturiser

Imagine you've mixed a foundation with your favourite moisturiser. That's exactly the coverage level you get with a tinted moisturiser if you prefer something lighter. Another hybrid product, it's a no-brainer if you want something that lightly hydrates and evens out your skin tone at the same time.

What is tinted moisturiser?

A tinted moisturiser is like a makeup triple treat: it will give you coverage, even skin tone and cover up redness. Think of it as a foundation, moisturiser and concealer skincare product all rolled into one handy tube. You can use a tinted moisturiser on its own as a base, or layer it with other makeup.

Benefits include hydration, sun protection (if it contains SPF) and minimal coverage – all with a subtle dash of colour. That said, while we're all about making life easier and multitasking, despite the name, don't relegate your usual moisturiser to the sidelines.

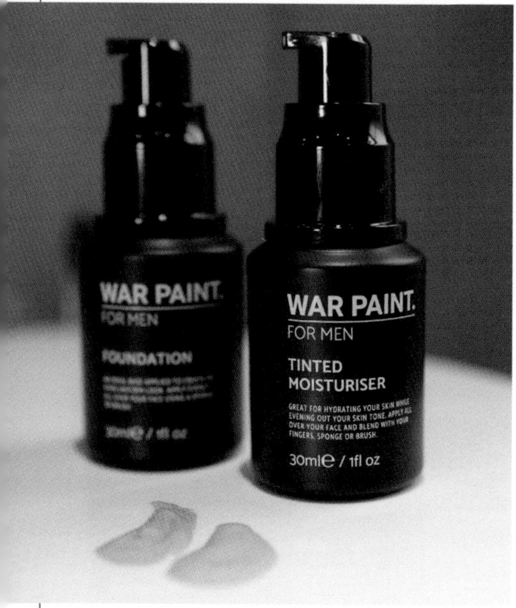

A tinted moisturiser has an element of hydration, but probably not enough that you can forego a dedicated moisturiser completely (especially in the winter months). If you have dehydrated skin, it's wise to double up.

Why use it?

If you like the idea of your skin showing through your base, a tinted moisturiser is a good option. Giving your skin an even finish, it's the kind of low-key product that will prompt your colleagues to comment on how 'healthy' you look without being able to quite put their finger on why.

Use it to cover up redness, mask blemishes and even make it look like you just got back from a weekend in Monaco. With a lower-level coverage than a foundation and a much lighter formulation, it blends effortlessly so you can apply it in the same way you would a moisturiser – perfect if you're short on time: just apply and go.

Tip

If you plan to be out in the sun all day long, the SPF in your tinted moisturiser probably isn't enough protection so first apply a layer of a higher SPF. Better to be safe than sorry, eh?

When to use tinted moisturiser

Find a tinted moisturiser in the right shade for your skin and you'll probably want to use it daily.

Once you've applied your skincare – and it's fully absorbed – a tinted moisturiser is your next step. Generally, it's a base product that is used on its own because it pretty much does everything besides giving you a high level of coverage. That's where foundation comes in....

Foundation vs tinted moisturiser

Can't decide between these two base leaders? If we were talking boxing weight class, a tinted moisturiser would be your lightweight contender and foundation is more like a heavyweight. If you feel more confident with stronger coverage on your skin, go for foundation.

Foundation is a thicker base that works on its own or alongside other products, while tinted moisturiser is thinner in texture so you can expect lighter coverage, but added hydration. Yes, tinted moisturiser can still conceal blemishes, but typically it won't cover major scars or heavy acne. Both products can be layered with concealer if you want extra reinforcement to cover up a spot that's out of control.

You shouldn't need to wear two products as a base simultaneously. But if you like the idea of switching between the two, think about going seasonal. Try a tinted moisturiser for a lighter base in the summer, and wear a foundation for more coverage in winter.

THE LOWDOWN:
BB/CC cream

Some tint bases fall into the alphabet-style category of BB or CC creams, but let's not overcomplicate things. If you see a label saying BB cream, it stands for 'blemish balm', aka a sheer tint that will help smooth and blur your skin. CC creams are similar but have additional colour-correcting properties.

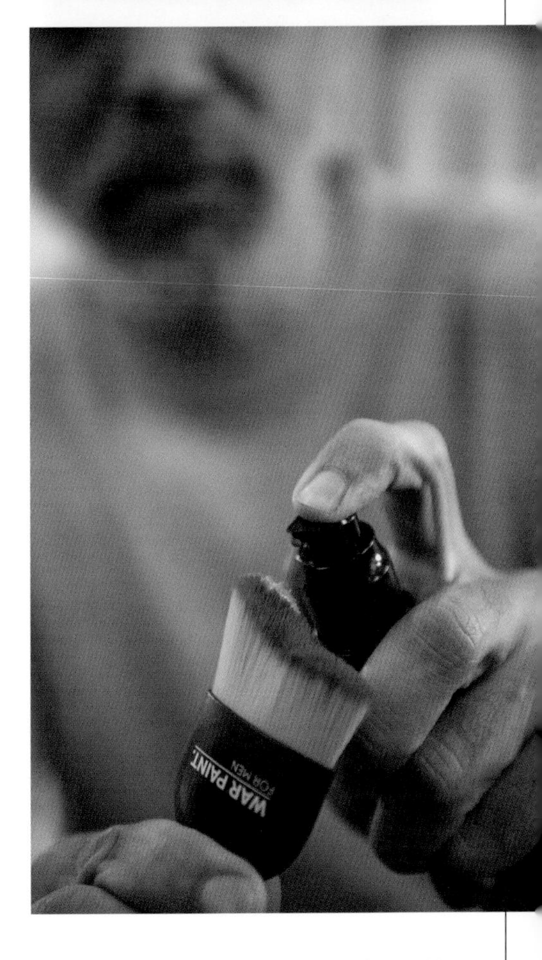

How to apply tinted moisturiser: Using your fingers

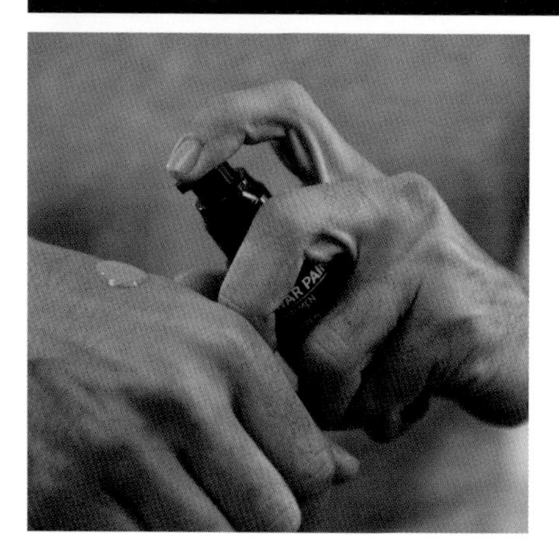

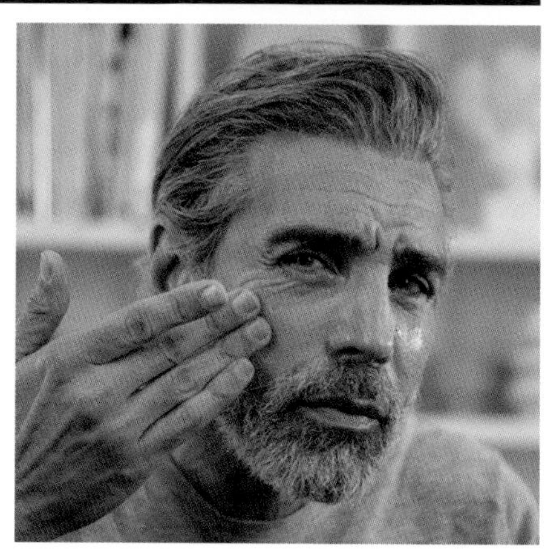

1 Pump a pea-sized amount of product on to the back of your hand and dab it on to your face.

2 Using your fingers, massage it into your whole face evenly, just like a normal moisturiser.

How to apply tinted moisturiser: Using a sponge

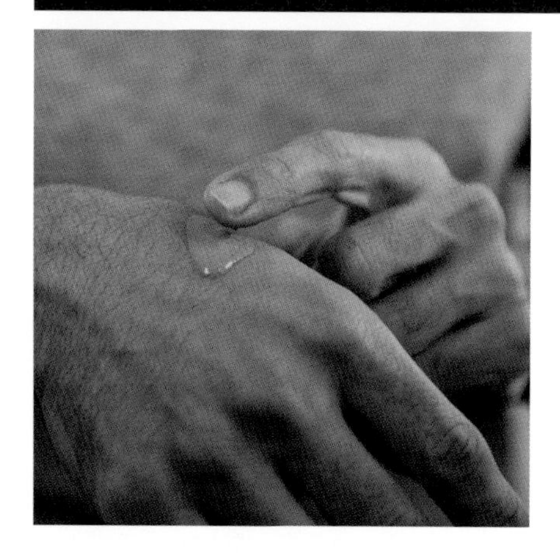

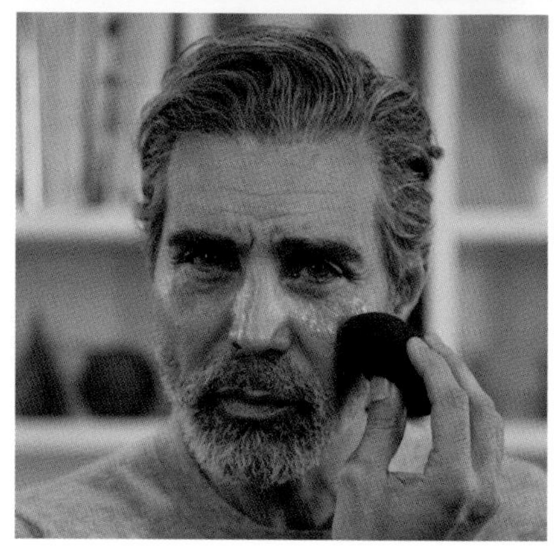

1 Dot the product on to the back of your hand using your fingertip so you can control the amount of product you're using.

2 With a damp sponge, blend in the product across the face. Dab rather than pull the sponge across your face for better results.

How to apply tinted moisturiser: Using a brush

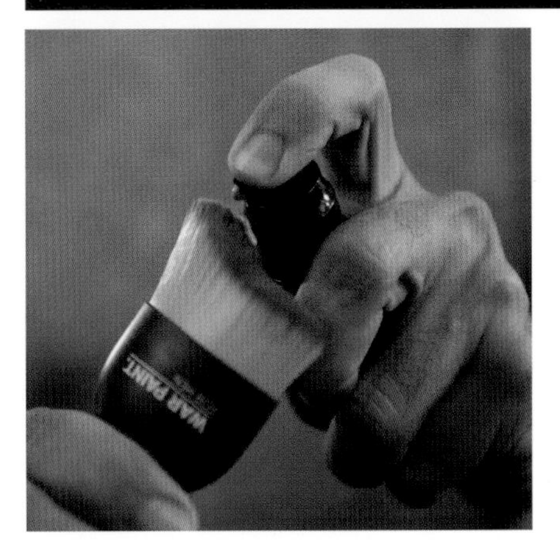

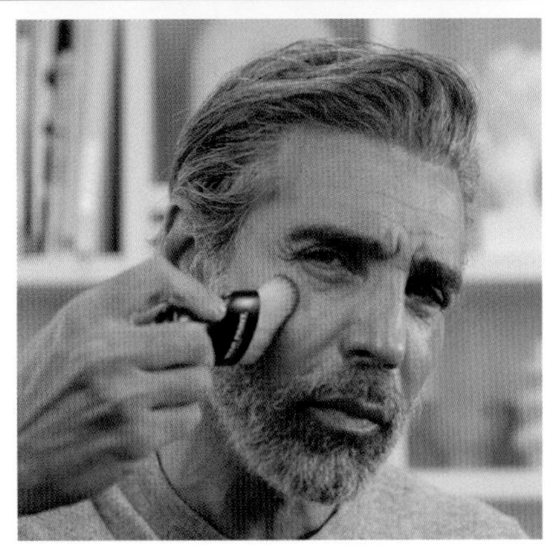

1 Dot the product directly on to your application brush.

2 Dab the brush on to your face to spread the product and blend it into your skin.

Do and don't

✓ Do skip the anti-shine powder. The whole point of tinted moisturiser is to look like you're not wearing any makeup.

✗ Don't forget to remove your tinted moisturiser at night.
It may be hydrating on the skin but the makeup element still always needs to be removed before bed so a) it doesn't damage your skin and b) it doesn't end up all over your pillowcase.

Scan to watch the **'How to apply tinted moisturiser'** video

Tip

Keep your skin type in mind when you're choosing a tinted moisturiser. If you're more prone to breakouts, look for an oil-free formula. If you have dry skin, look for one that maximises hydration.

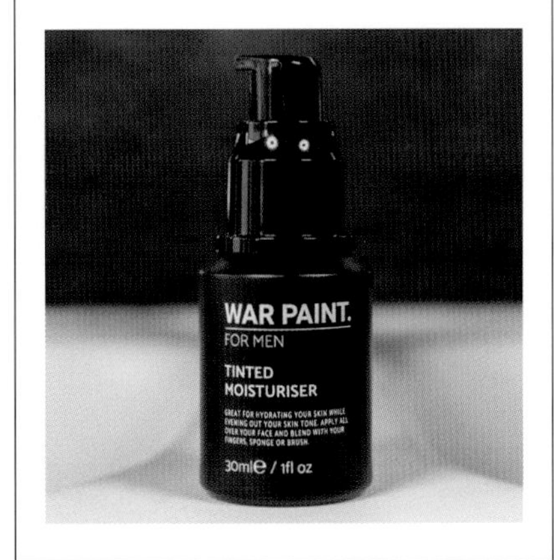

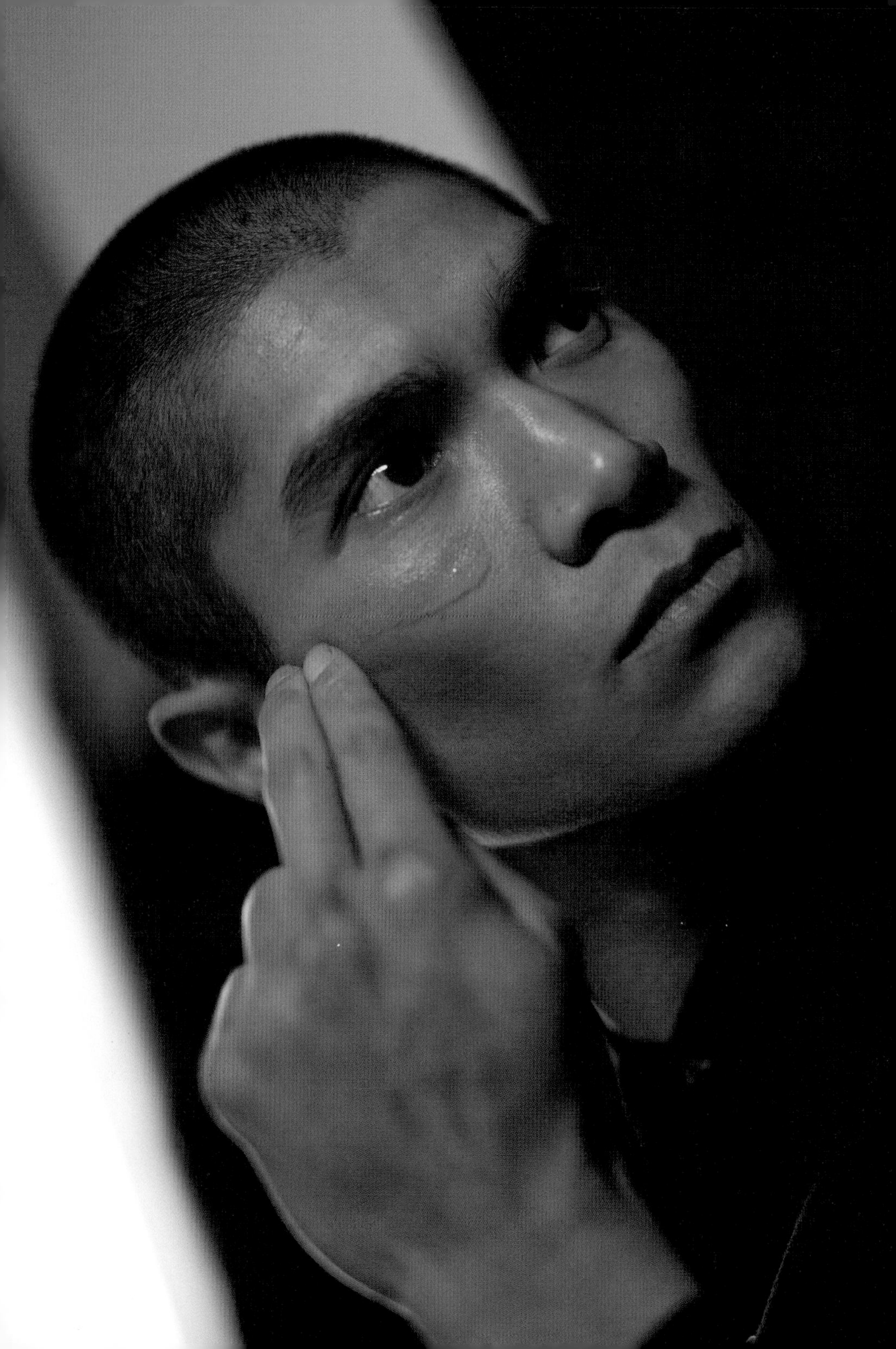

Foundation

Foundation is your go-to if you want that extra bit of coverage. Apply it to your face (and neck) to give your complexion an even, uniform colour, cover any flaws, and boost your skin confidence. Literally acting as the 'foundation' for your makeup, it also allows you to easily layer products on top.

What is foundation?

Coming in liquid, powder and even stick form, foundation is a neutral-toned base that evens out any skin imperfections and gives you a consistent colour. For a no-makeup makeup look, go lightweight and matte so that you can build up the coverage easily.

Steer clear of foundations that are labelled as 'illuminating' or 'brightening', which usually translates as, um, subtle shimmer. Anything touted as 'dewy' should also be avoided as this can exaggerate the shine on men's oil-prone skin.

Why use it?

If a tinted moisturiser or BB cream isn't quite hitting the spot when it comes to your base, it could be time to graduate to foundation. With a thicker formulation, a foundation will give you much more coverage – ideal if you have blemishes or hyperpigmentation that a sheer tint might struggle with.

A foundation can vary in coverage (how much pigment it contains), from light and sheer to high and full. Sticking to a light-to-medium coverage with a matte finish is ideal for the most natural look. Beware: heavy, long-wear foundations can be tricky to blend in so always pick a lightweight, buildable formula that's easy to work with. You can always apply more product if it's needed.

When to use foundation

Provided that you cleanse properly, there's no time limit on how regularly you put on your foundation, whether it's seven days a week or the occasional base for a big night out.

Primer isn't a must, but applying it before your foundation will give it some extra staying power. To really ace your base, apply the foundation to your whole face and neck and blend well so it looks undetectable on your skin. Fingers, sponge or brush – the application method you use is down to you.

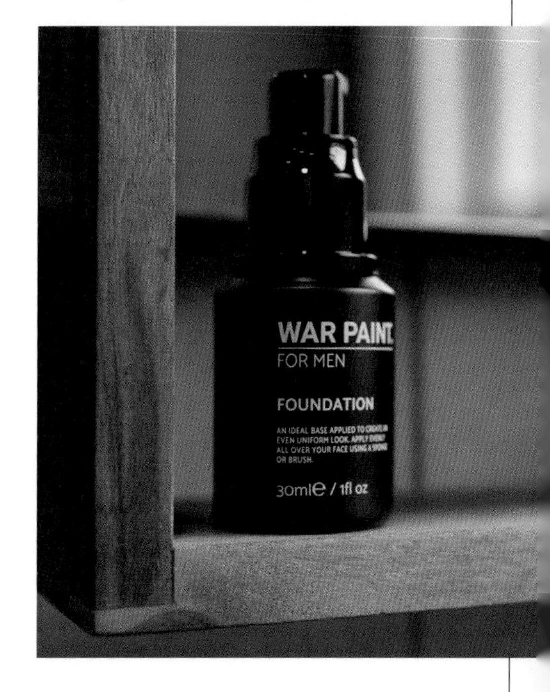

Post-foundation products

We get it, makeup can be confusing. Can you wear it solo? In what order do you apply your products? Foundation can be worn solo if you're after an even, perfected finish. But it doesn't stop there. These three products can all be used *after* you put your tube of foundation down.

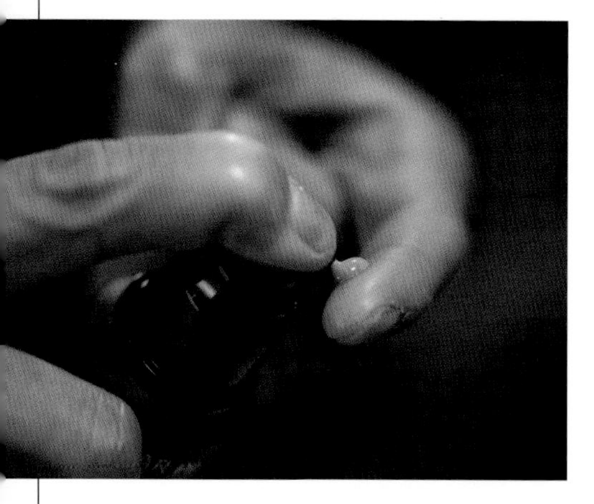

- Concealer to cover imperfections: yup, your concealer can be used after a base of foundation has been applied, to cover up any blemishes or dark circles that are still visible.
- Bronzer for a dash of colour: if you feel like your complexion is almost too even after applying foundation, add colour back in with bronzer and pretend you've been to Barbados (or Bognor Regis, depending on how subtle you go).
- Anti-shine to mattify your face: don't panic if you've applied foundation and you still have unwanted shine. Lightly brush on some mattifying anti-shine powder, focusing on your T-zone (see page 82).

How to apply foundation: Using your fingers

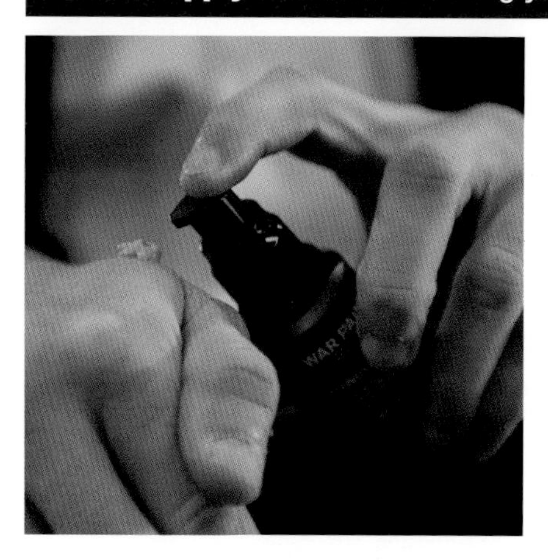

1 Dot some product on to your face using your fingertips.

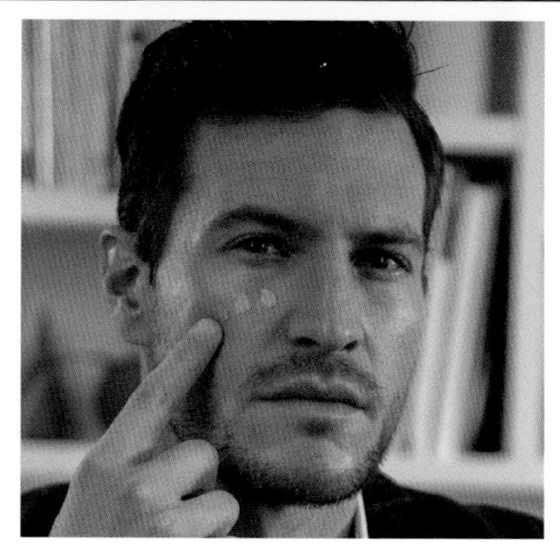

2 Use your fingers to evenly blend in the product across your face in all areas, including the upper part of the neck, so the colour is uniform.

Testing, testing – how to find the right shade for you

Yup, application is important but finding the right shade is key to getting that natural finish we all want. Here are our hacks for matching up the tone to your skin so nobody will notice.

- Avoid testing a shade on your arm, wrist or back of your hand. If you can, try it out on your jawline to get the most accurate match.
- Swipe three shades on your jawline, wait ten minutes and then check in the mirror or take a selfie. The foundation that looks invisible is the right tone for you.
- Skip the in-store fluorescent lighting and always check out foundation in natural daylight to get the most accurate shade.

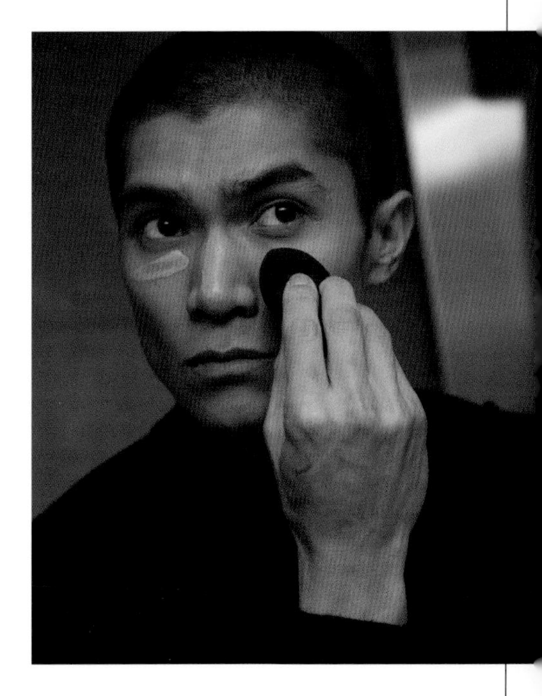

- It might sound obvious, but always test a foundation shade on your bare face, not over the top of existing makeup.
- Try to avoid wearing fake tan when you're sampling shades, unless you have it on the majority of the time.
- Your skin tone can change in warmer weather or after a vacation. You can either adjust the depth of your foundation, or mix in your usual shade with a darker colour during the summer months, to create your own bespoke shade.

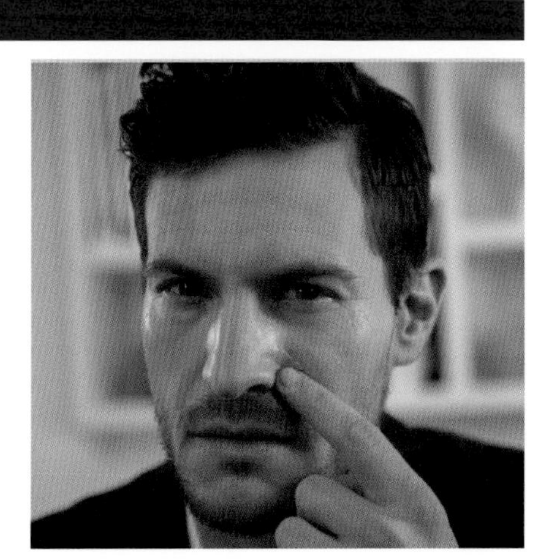

3 Use your finger to dab in any excess and smooth out trickier places, such as the creases of your nose.

Tip

Believe it or not, good foundation application doesn't finish at your face. Continue blending the product lightly on your neck and below your beard area and you'll create a more natural look.

How to apply foundation: Using a sponge

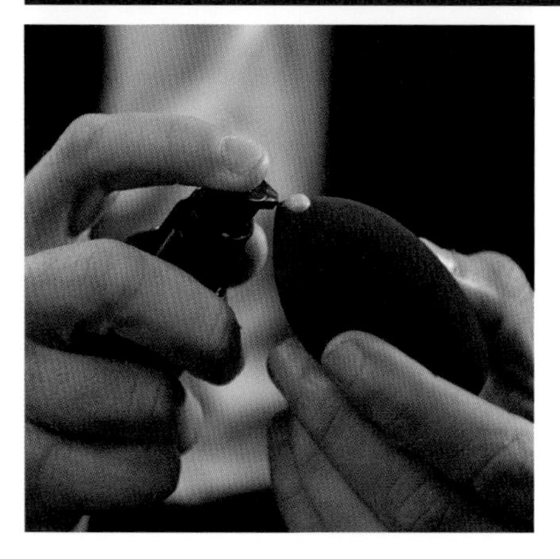

1 Dot the foundation evenly on to your face using the tip of the sponge.

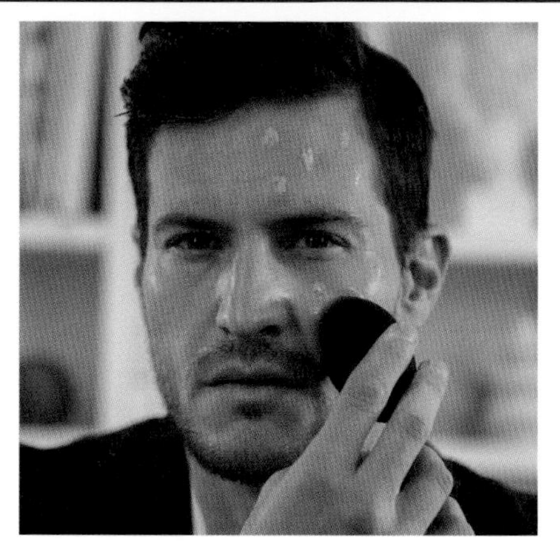

2 Using a damp sponge, blend in the product across the face using a dabbing motion rather than dragging it across your face.

How to apply foundation: Using a brush

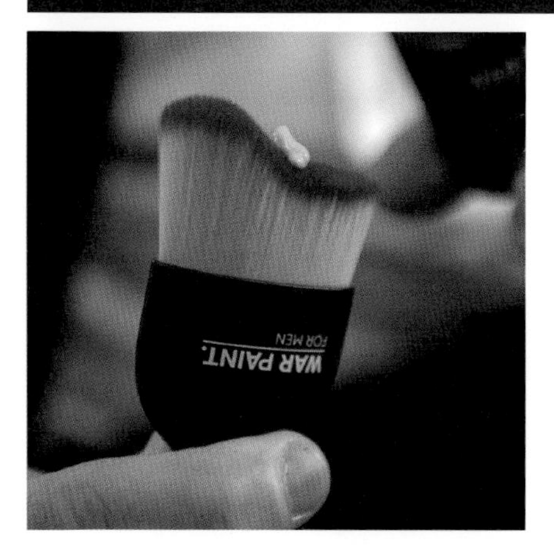

1 Dot a small, pea-sized amount of foundation on to your application brush.

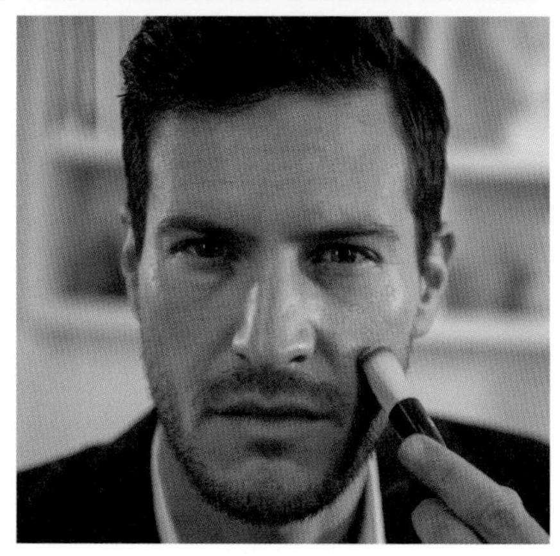

2 Use the brush to apply the foundation evenly across your face to fully blend it into the skin.

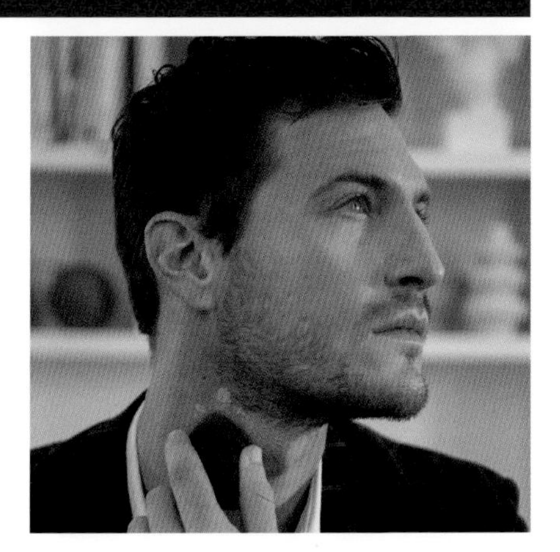

3 Make sure your face and neck match by blending the foundation into the top of your neck.

Tip

Pay extra attention to your beard/stubble zone so you don't have telltale uneven coverage. Dot foundation on the skin around your beard and then dab it using the edge of a damp sponge. You can always use a beard brush to remove any build-up in facial hair and eyebrows.

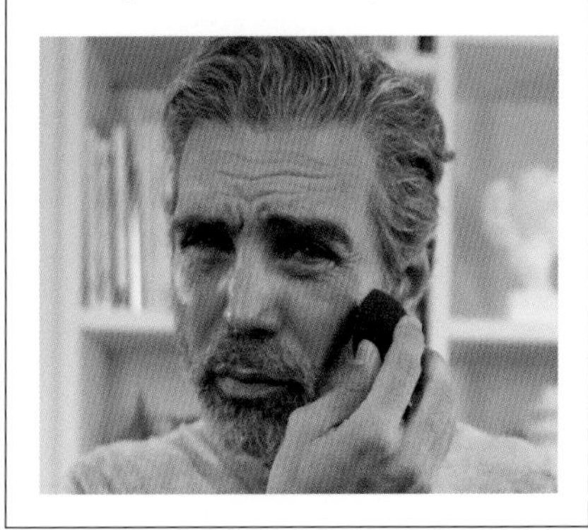

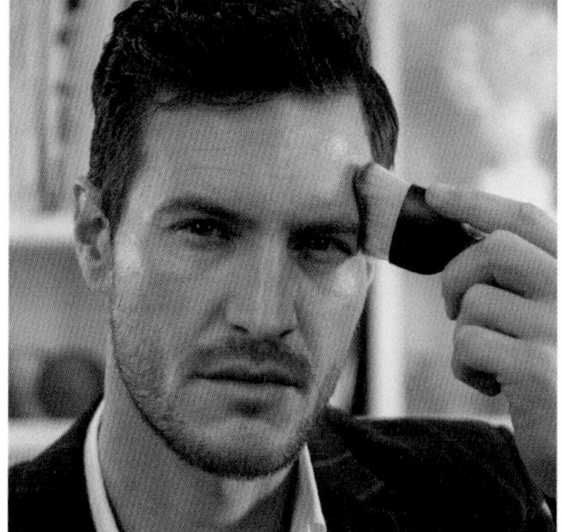

3 Repeat and apply more foundation if needed, ensuring that you don't load up the brush with too much product.

Do and don't

✓ Do go easy with the amount of product. A dot of foundation can go a long way so start off with a small amount and build up the coverage. You can always add more if you feel like your skin needs it.

✗ Don't choose a shade that's too light or dark for your skin tone. You don't want your face to look a different colour to the rest of your body.

Scan to watch the **'How to apply foundation'** step-by-step video

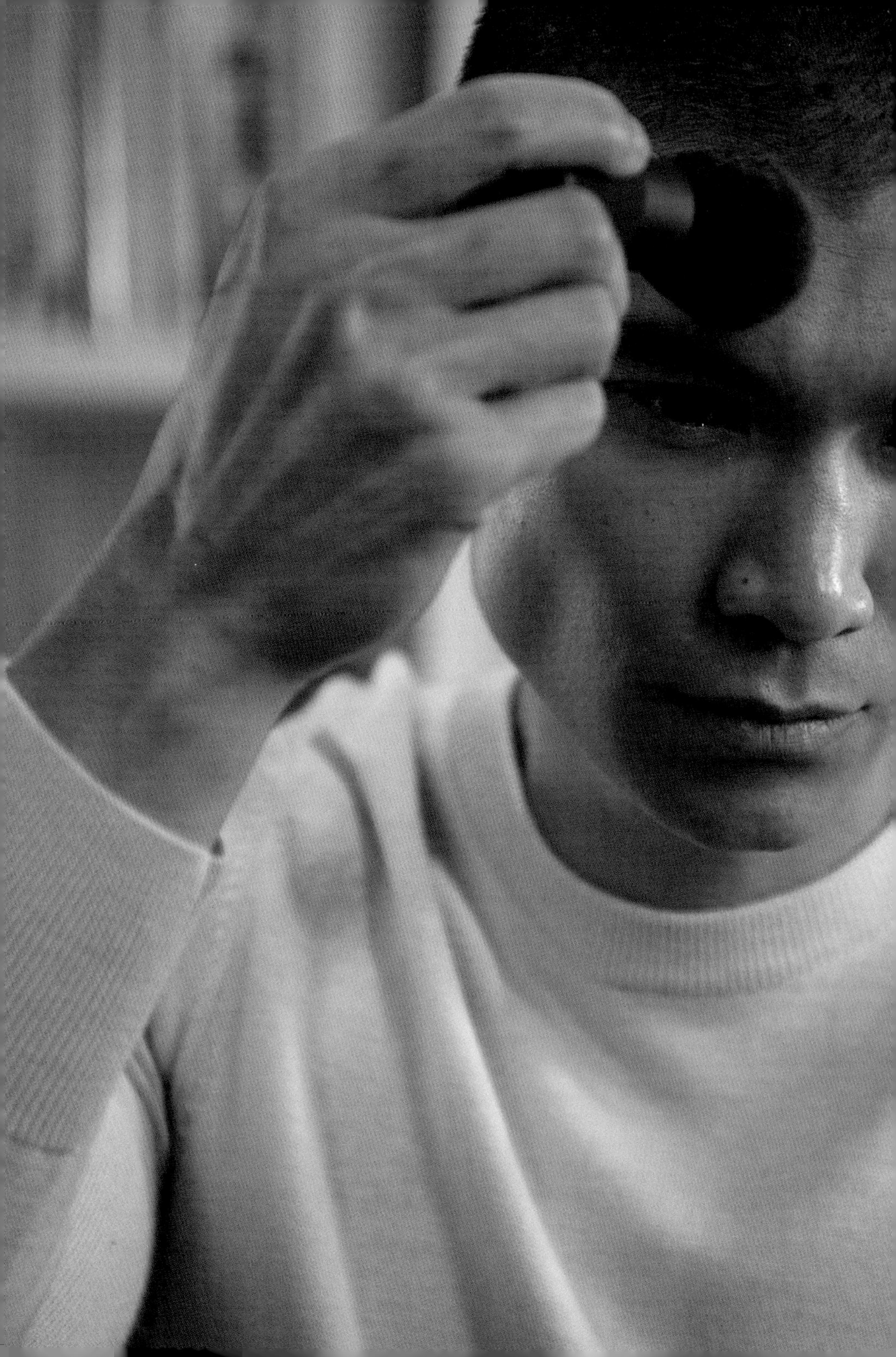

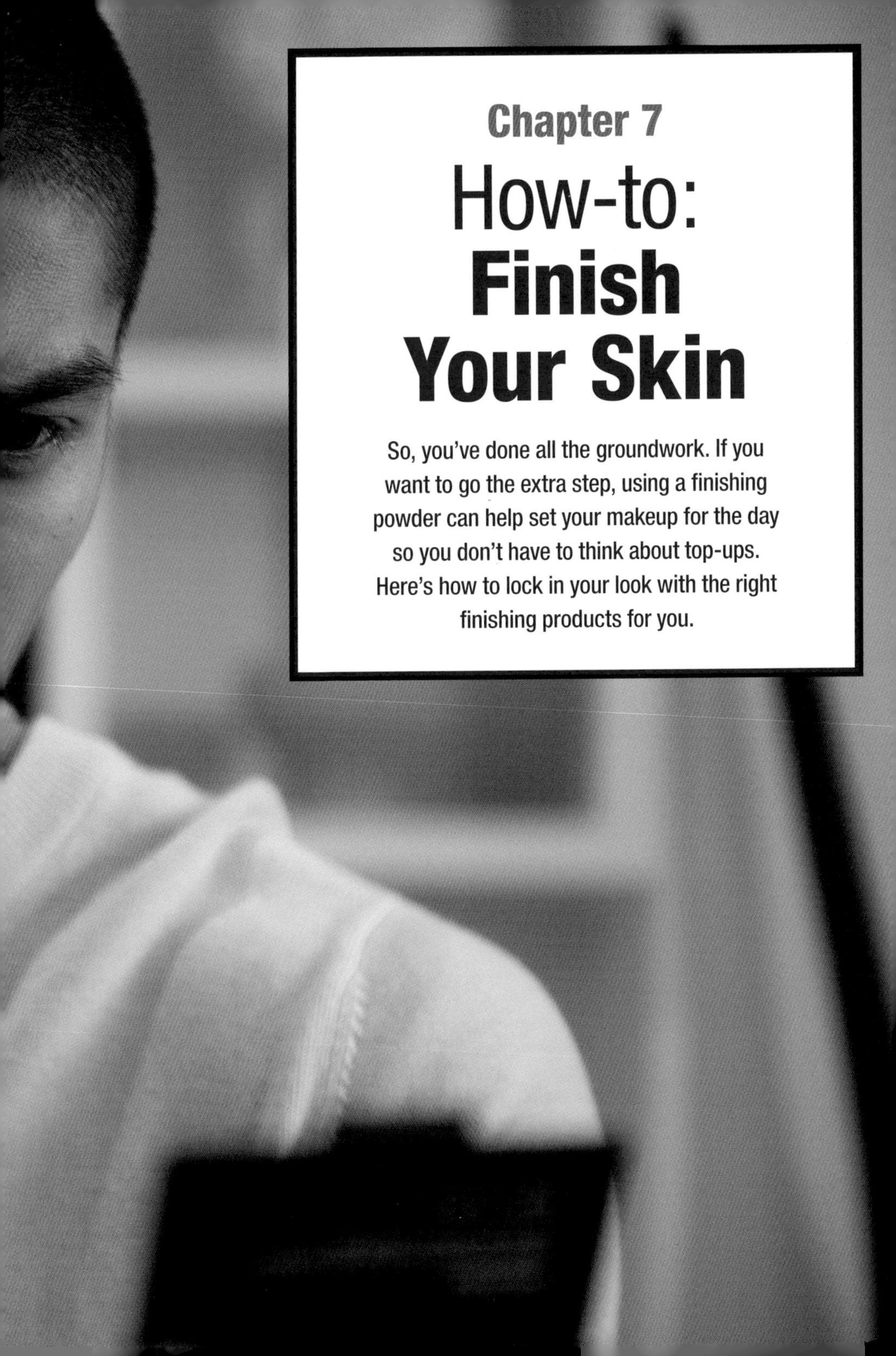

Chapter 7

How-to: **Finish Your Skin**

So, you've done all the groundwork. If you want to go the extra step, using a finishing powder can help set your makeup for the day so you don't have to think about top-ups. Here's how to lock in your look with the right finishing products for you.

Anti-shine powder

If you're prone to oily or greasy-looking skin, become best mates with an anti-shine powder. It gives you a matte finish in seconds. As the name suggests, this game-changing powder helps do away with excess grease and shine. Result.

Why use anti-shine powder?

A good anti-shine powder not only puts a stop to a relentless sweaty brow, but it also helps prevent unwanted shine because it mops up excess oils. Clever. It's a quick-fix product if you want matte-looking skin in 30 seconds. Plus, shiny skin rarely holds makeup well so it creates extra staying power, too.

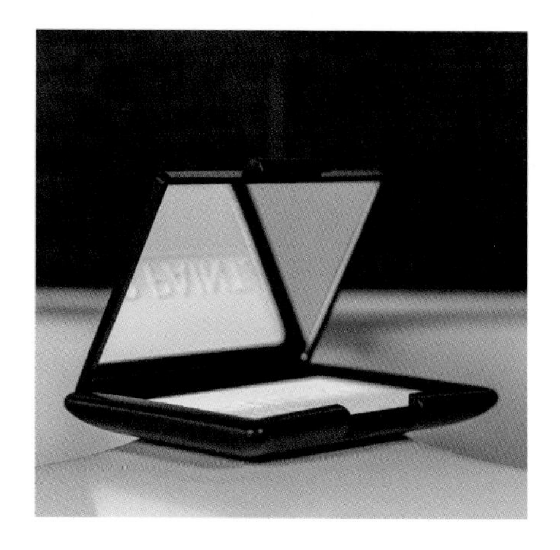

How to apply anti-shine powder

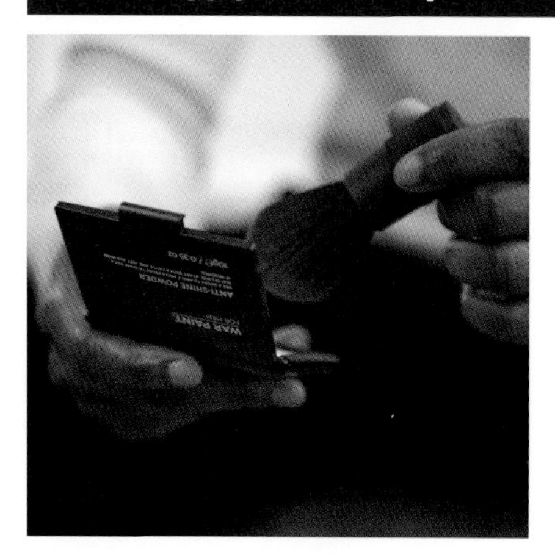

1 Take a small amount of anti-shine powder using a powder brush.

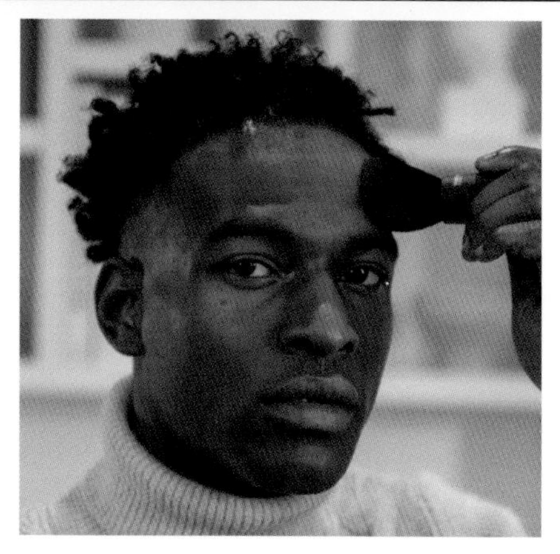

2 Apply it all over your face in light, circular motions or just stick to the obvious oily zones.

Can you see it?

Nope, anti-shine pressed powder is usually translucent, so you can't see it on. That doesn't mean that you can't go overboard, though. If you notice that the powder is making you look pale then you've probably used too much. Give it a few practice runs to see what works for your skin.

When do I use it?

Anti-shine powder is a great product to use to finish off your makeup routine, so apply it as the very last step. As we always say, there are no hard-and-fast rules though, so you can use it solo for a matte, shine-free look if you just want a quick fix. This product also doubles up as a setting powder. Don't be confused by the latter, it just helps your products to stay put for longer. Win-win.

Tip

If shine is a persistent problem and you're feeling self-conscious, carry blotting papers in your pocket when you're on the go. They will mop up excess oil in seconds and won't mess up your makeup.

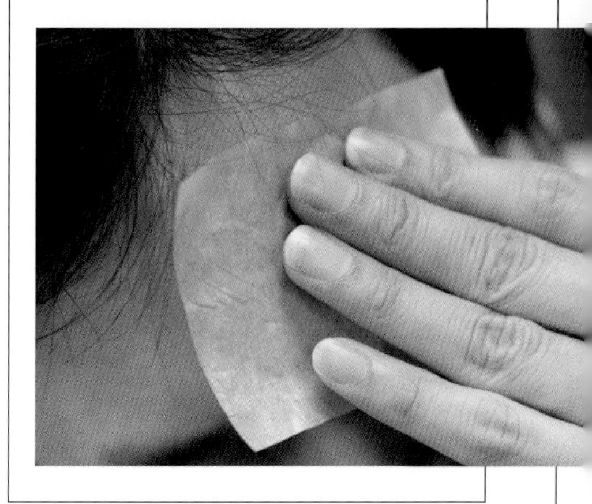

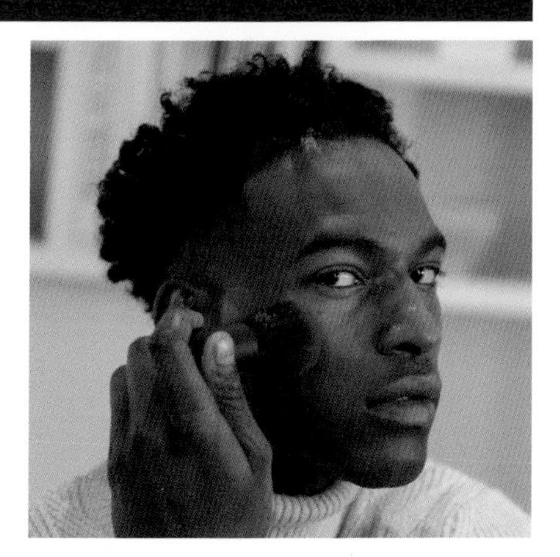

3 If needed, add a little more powder to the oilier areas of your face.

Do and don't

✓ Do work on each area for a few seconds to absorb all excess oil, then move on to the next area. You can always go back to apply more powder if needed.

✗ Don't rub the skin. Always gently brush on the powder. If you're wearing a base, rubbing the brush over your skin will remove it and you'll have to reapply.

Scan to watch the **'How to apply anti-shine powder'** video

Keeping oily skin under control

Why so greasy?

Hands up if you look in the mirror at lunchtime and your face is shinier than a Christmas tree bauble. We've all been there. And if you suffer with persistently greasy skin, it can make you feel like other people can see it from outer space.

Let's get down to the nitty-gritty of why we get greasy skin. It turns out you can blame male genetics. Not only is a guy's skin about 23% thicker than a woman's, but men also have larger pores to boot. This means that we naturally produce about four times more oil than a woman's skin, resulting in that unwanted shine.

The bad news: oil production in men's skin doesn't slow down as we get older. The good news: we *can* control it.

Do and don't

✓ Do always wash your face after you exercise. This is crucial for removing unwanted dirt and sweat that can cause breakouts.

✗ Don't take hot showers – they can make your skin very dry, which in turn leads to an oilier face. Take cooler showers or aim to reduce the temperature of the water towards the end of your shower, especially if you're washing your face.

THE LOWDOWN:
The T-zone

Greasy hotspots you should know about? Your T-zone is the oiliest area on your face. Shaped like a T (it would be weird if it wasn't), it starts from the mid-point and sides of your forehead and extends down your face, including the sides of the nose and centre of your chin.

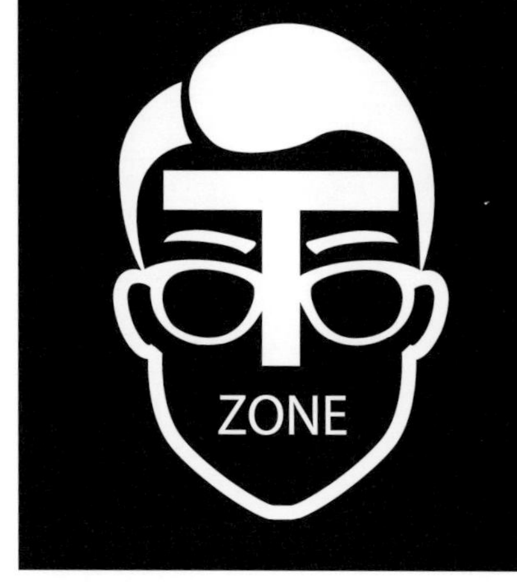

How to prevent shiny-looking skin

From shifting your everyday skin prep to mattifying makeup, you can help to halt the greasy look (trust us). What shiny skin needs is a double-pronged approach: gentle skincare to treat it, and fine-particle makeup to disguise its effects. That's where your anti-shine powder comes in.

Aim to wash and cleanse your face twice a day to eliminate blackheads and dirt and keep pores unclogged. Using a gentle exfoliator will also help to keep up cell turnover. It sounds backwards, but if your skin's mega-oily, it might seem like moisturising is the opposite of what you'd want to do, but often excess moisture occurs because your face is over-compensating for dehydrated skin. The solution? Hydrate regularly with a light and oil-free moisturiser so your face isn't producing that excess oil.

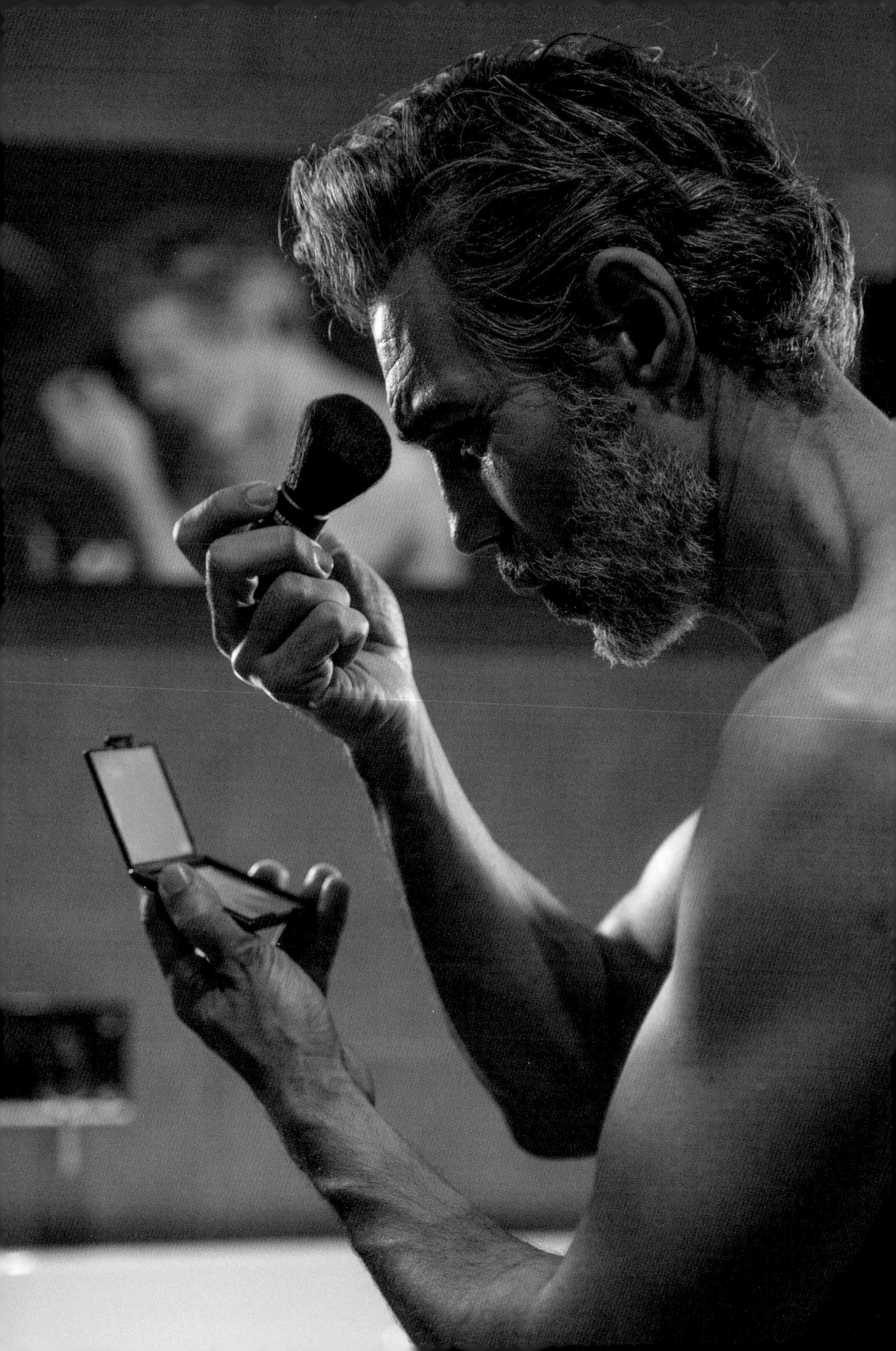

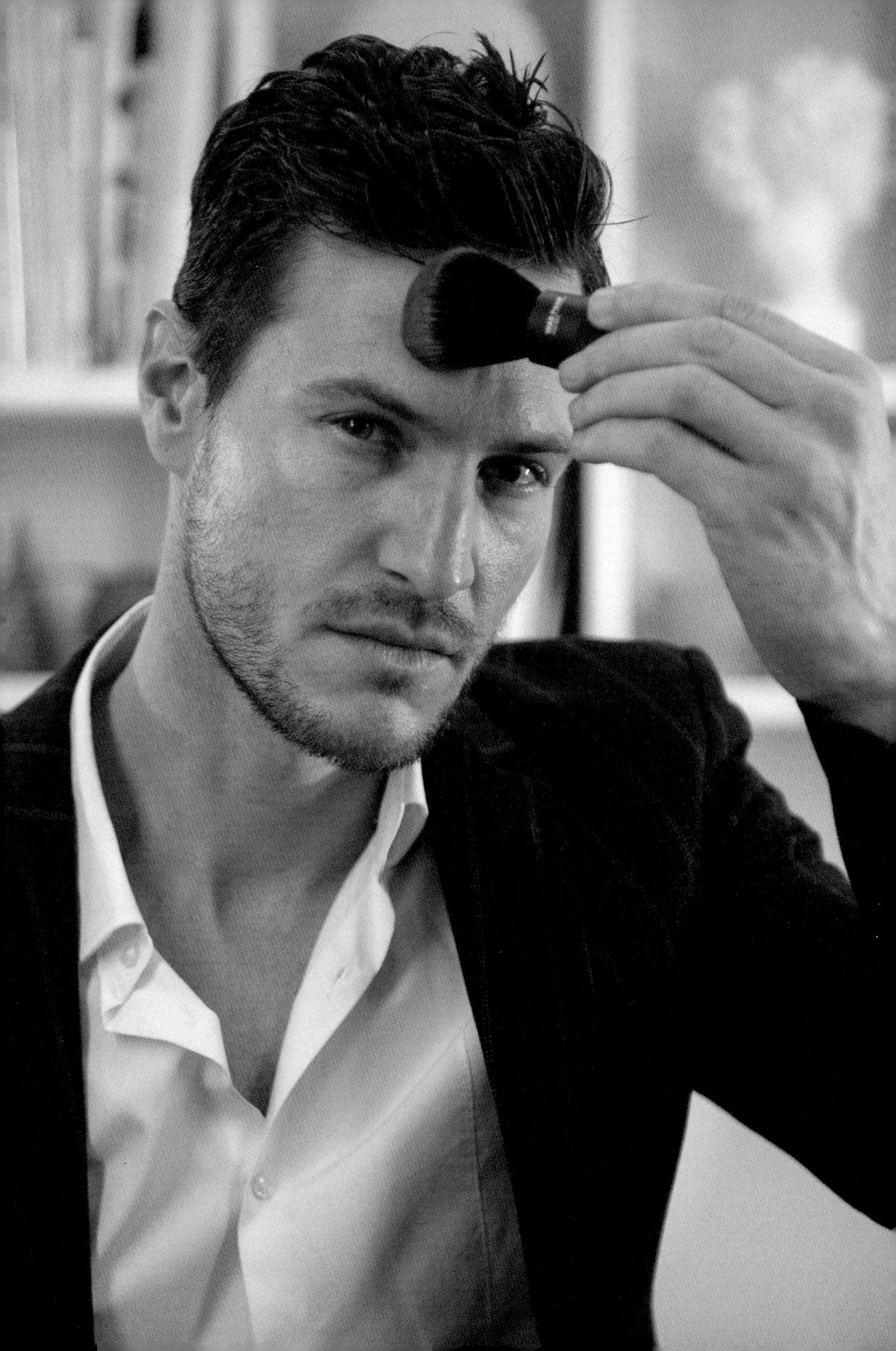

Bronzing powder

No sun, no problem, because bronzer will always have your back. From subtle to defined, it gives you the appearance of a suntan in 20 seconds flat. Think of it as the pale-skin saviour of your kit bag.

Bronzing 101

Q: What is bronzer?
A: A good bronzer will add some instant, healthy colour to your face, especially in the winter months. To make your bronzer look as realistic as possible, focus on the areas where the sun would naturally hit your face, such as temples and cheekbones.

Q: Can you get different types?
A: Yes, you can get powder or liquid bronzers. Powders are probably the most versatile formulation for men's skin because you can build up the colour easily using a powder brush. Our advice? Avoid anything that isn't matte. Men's skin is already prone to shine so any hint of shimmer won't be a good idea. Liquid bronzers are a cool option if you want an all-over hint of colour – mix a dot with your usual moisturiser for a subtle result and build up from there.

Q: What can it be used with?
A: Because bronzer is a finishing product, it can be used alongside most makeup, such as foundation, tinted moisturiser and concealer. Just brush a little bronzer over the top of your base to give yourself a tanned look and wait for the 'have you been away?' questions to roll in.

Q: When should I apply bronzer?
A: Make it one of the last finishing products you apply in your routine – so after your foundation, tinted moisturiser or concealer. Bronzer is usually the last step before you head off for work or that big night out.

THE LOWDOWN:
The figure 3 move

Mimicking the figure 3 is an easy way for beginners to get their bronzer on point. Start at the top of your forehead just over your temple, bring the brush down and under your cheekbone, then back again to the hairline and out under the jawline, as if you're outlining a figure 3. Repeat on the other side.

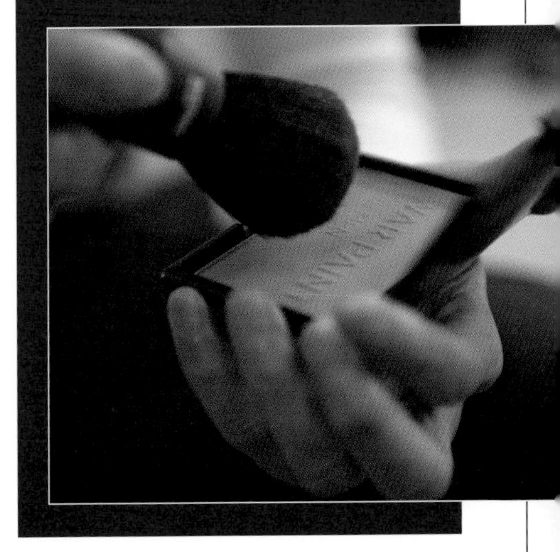

How to apply bronzer: The natural look

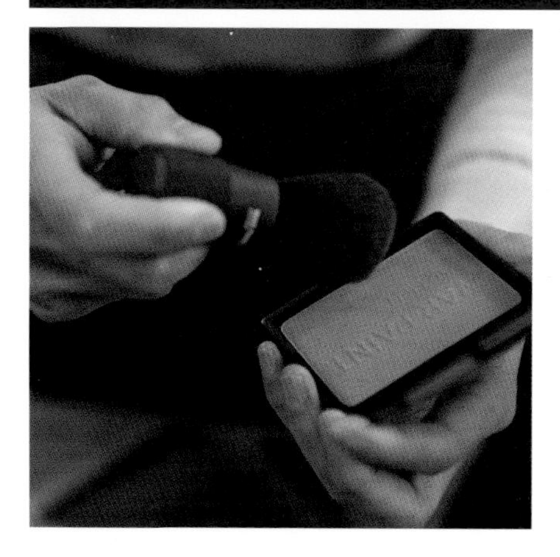

1 Take a small amount of bronzer using a powder brush and blow or tap off any excess.

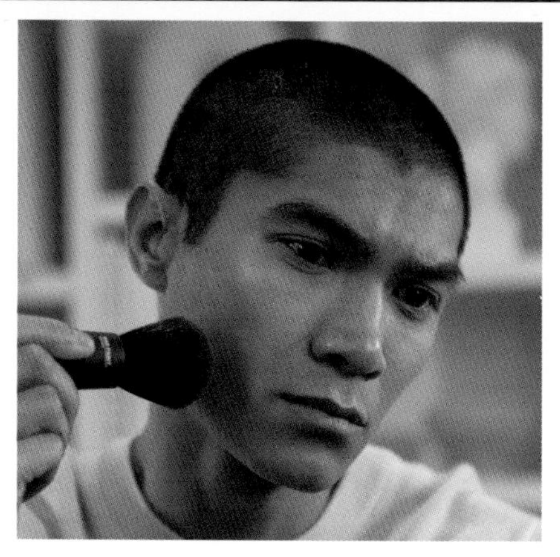

2 Lightly sweep the brush in a figure 3 motion, starting from your temples, coming in under your cheekbone and finishing on your jawline.

How to apply bronzer: The defined look

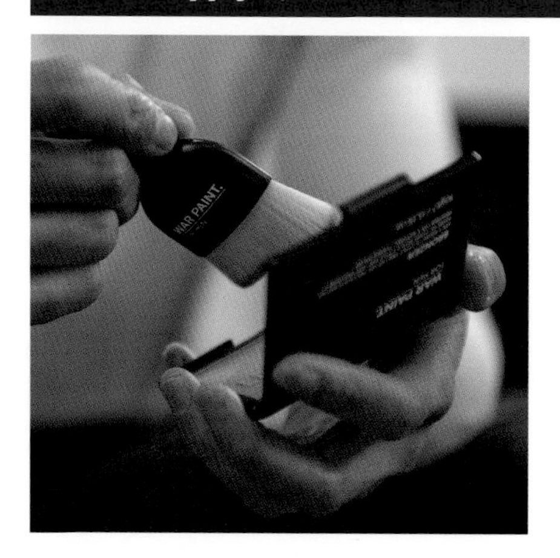

1 Take a small amount of bronzer using an application brush and tap off any excess.

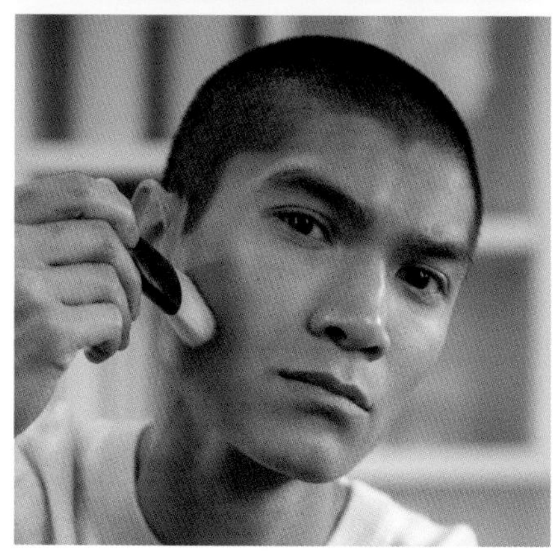

2 Sweep the brush across the tops of your forehead and under your cheekbones and jawline.

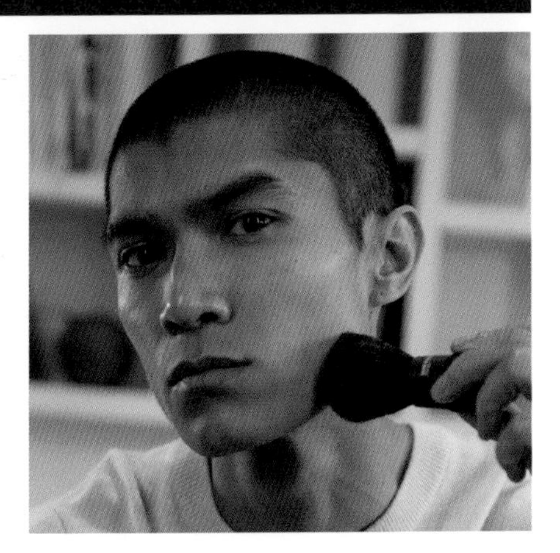

3 Repeat the figure 3 motion on the other side of your face.

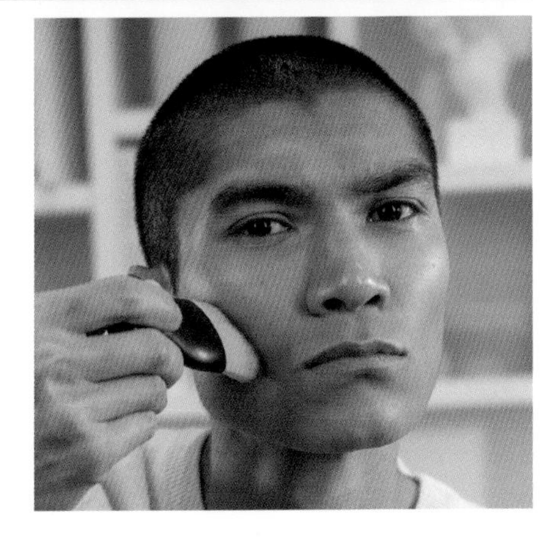

3 Repeat to build up the desired darker colour.

Tip

Switching up your brush will dictate your level of colour. For a natural look, go for a powder brush with a fluffy texture. To go more defined, try a denser application brush.

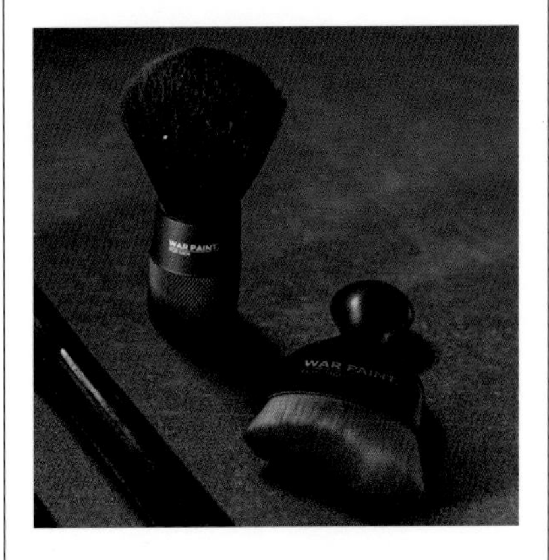

Do and don't

✓ Do also apply a light layer of bronzer to the rest of your face and neck so your face doesn't look too dark compared to your neck colour.

✗ Don't ignore the lines of your face. Allow the brush to follow the higher planes of your face – temples, cheekbones and jawline (where the sun would naturally hit) to get a natural-look bronze.

Scan to watch the **'How to apply bronzer'** step-by-step video

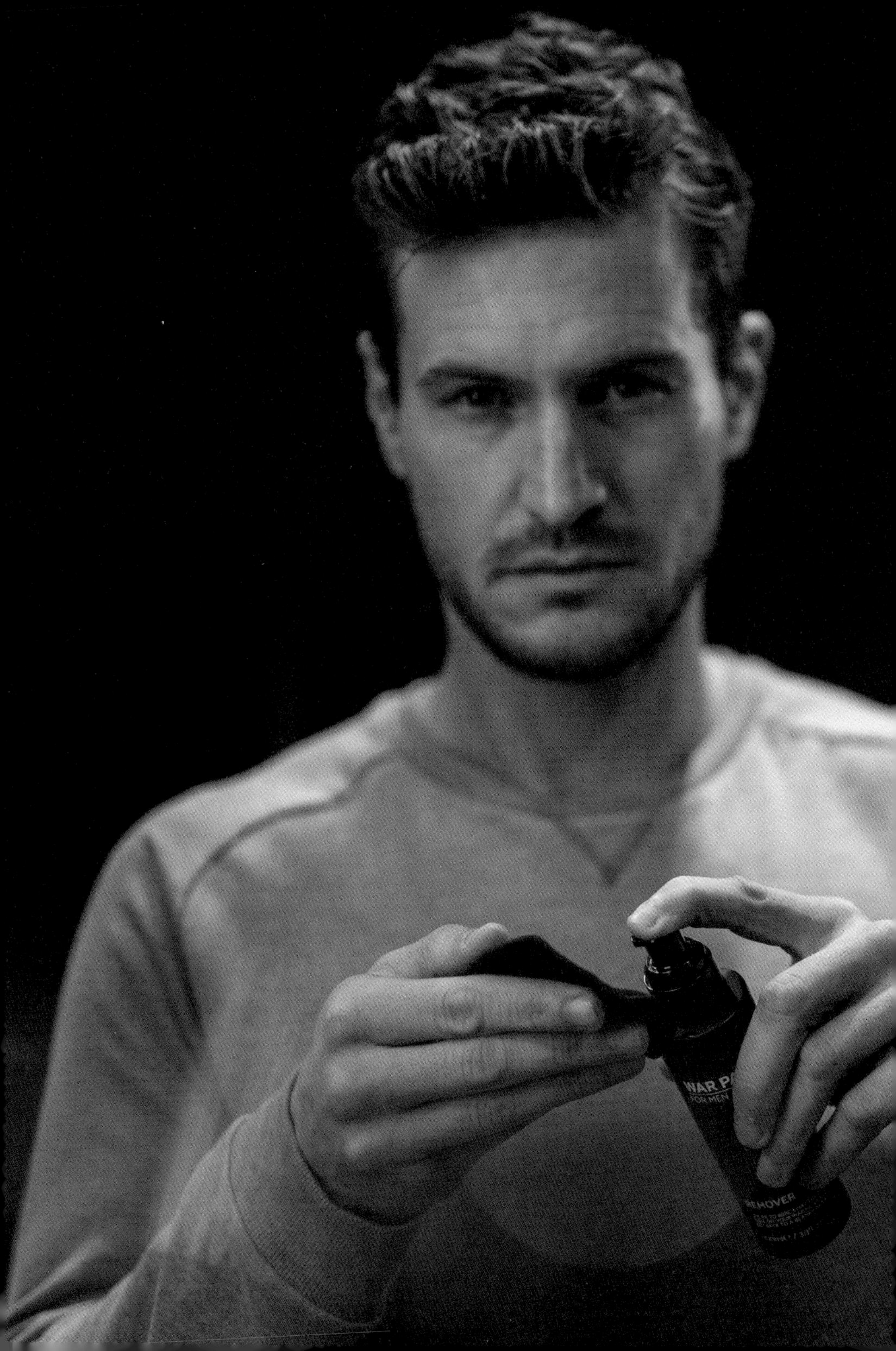
FOR MEN

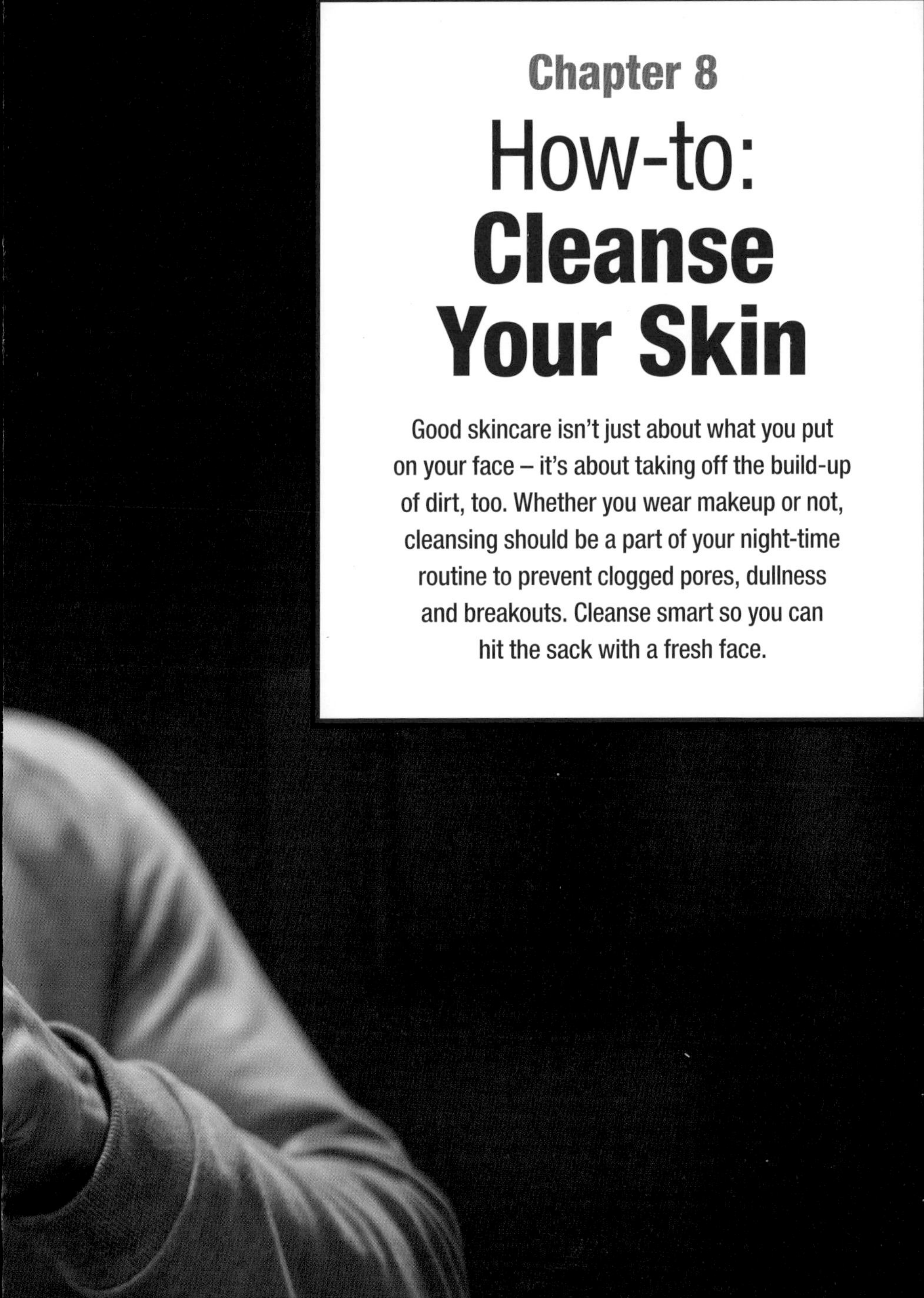

Chapter 8

How-to: Cleanse Your Skin

Good skincare isn't just about what you put on your face – it's about taking off the build-up of dirt, too. Whether you wear makeup or not, cleansing should be a part of your night-time routine to prevent clogged pores, dullness and breakouts. Cleanse smart so you can hit the sack with a fresh face.

How to cleanse your skin

Granted, it's never going to be the most exciting part of your day, but cleansing is a daily habit that's wise to adopt for well-behaved skin – whether you're wearing makeup or not. How you cleanse is down to your skin type and standard routine. Get it right and cleansing shouldn't feel like a chore.

Why cleanse?

A bar of body soap just won't cut it when it comes to cleansing your face properly. At best, it will dry out your skin. At worst, you can expect irritation and redness, especially if you have sensitive skin.

Using a cleanser that's specifically engineered for the face will help deep-clean your pores and remove any debris that might lead to breakouts or other skin issues. Leave your face uncleansed and you could be spending the night with dead skin cells and other impurities that have transferred to your pillow.

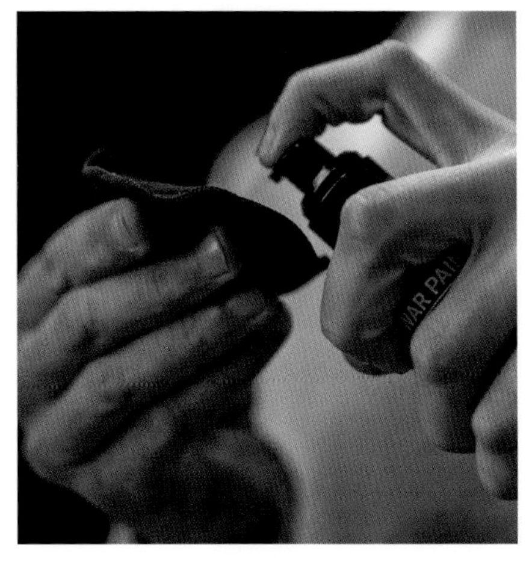

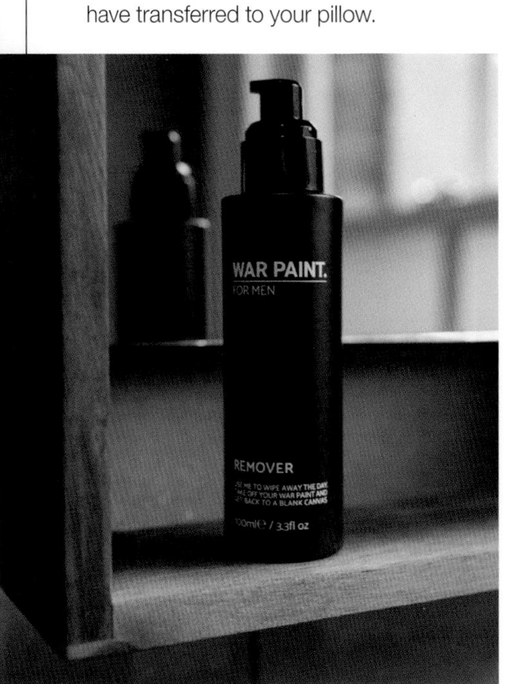

How often?

Cleansing daily is the goal to prevent clogged pores and dull skin. It's a step you should never skip – no matter how many pints you've sunk. Conversely, washing your face more than once a day can dry out some skin types so try to establish a routine that works for you. A morning cleanse can therefore be optional, but cleansing before bed is mandatory since it will remove the daily build-up of dirt and grime. Another serious case for the pre-bedtime cleanse: you should never sleep in makeup.

If you want to freshen up in between cleanses, splash cool or lukewarm water on your face without going through the whole cleansing regime. Try to avoid using hot water as it can dry out your skin.

Which cleanser?

Your skin type is all-important when it comes to choosing the cleanser that's going to be most effective for your face. Just like moisturiser, cleansing isn't one size fits all; it needs to be tailored to your skin type, be it oily, dry, sensitive or combination. You've found the right one if it gently cleanses your skin without drying it out or causing any irritation.

Here's a quick breakdown to make life easier (check our skin type guide on page 47 if you're not sure).

- **IF YOU HAVE DRY SKIN**
  Cleanse your face with a cleansing cream or oil for an extra hit of hydration.

- **IF YOU HAVE NORMAL SKIN**
  A foaming gentle cleanser is ideal if you have 'regular', well-behaved skin – especially if you're down for cleansing twice a day.

- **IF YOU HAVE OILY/COMBINATION SKIN**
  Clarifying cleansers are well suited to oilier complexions as they help to control excess oil production and keep your skin balanced.

- **IF YOU HAVE ACNE-PRONE SKIN**
  Go for a cleanser that includes ingredients specifically geared towards preventing breakouts, such as salicylic acid, glycolic acid or benzoyl peroxide.

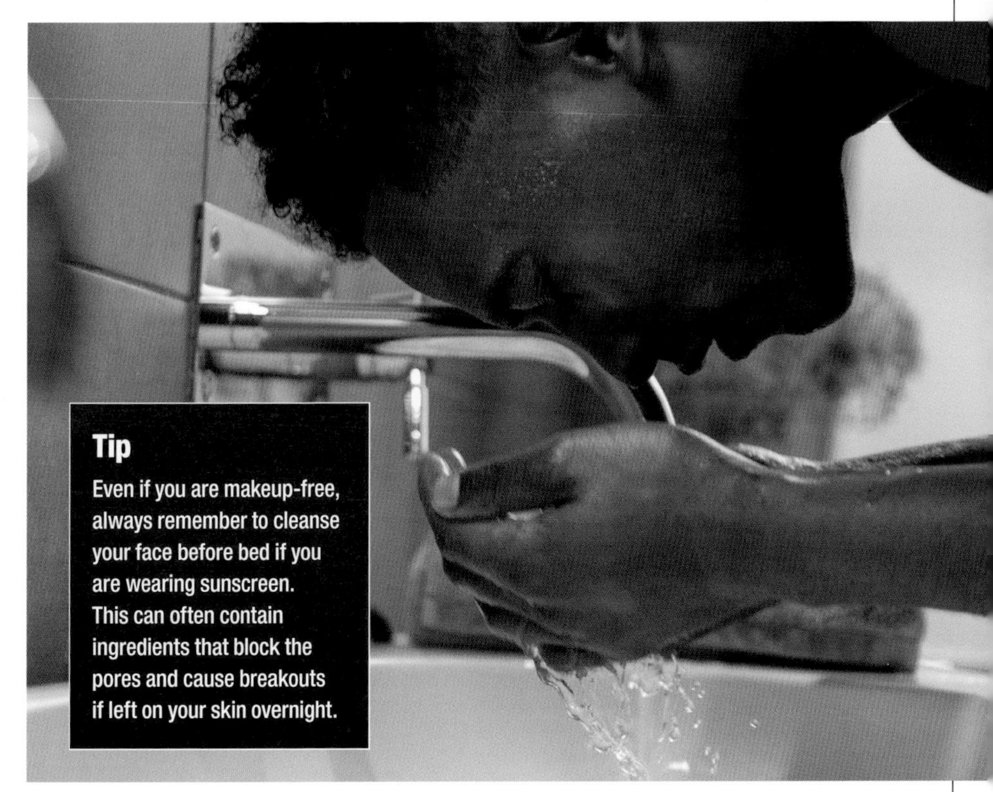

Tip

Even if you are makeup-free, always remember to cleanse your face before bed if you are wearing sunscreen. This can often contain ingredients that block the pores and cause breakouts if left on your skin overnight.

Levels of cleansing

With so many ways to cleanse, the best approach is to find a cleansing product that works for your skin type, but also your individual routine. Some of you might want a quick 20-second cleanse in the shower, others may feel that their skin needs a more thorough, deeper cleanse. Go with whatever fits in with your lifestyle and you're way more likely to stick to it.

The rapid cleanse: 30 seconds

Hey, it's OK if you want to be in and out of the bathroom in record time. Cleansing shouldn't feel like an extra chore on your skincare to-do list so choose a daily facial wash that's speedy but effective. Use it in the shower and the warm mist will encourage deeper exfoliation and unclog your pores, so you save time and water, and get a deeper cleanse to boot.

The power cleanse: 1 minute

Up your cleansing game with a gadget (any excuse, right?). A rechargeable facial cleansing brush that's specifically engineered for men's skin can oscillate at a frequency that produces hundreds of movements per second. Combined with a foaming gel cleanser, the brush's flexing action helps loosen dirt and oil and remove impurities from your pores. Just focus the brush on your forehead and nose for the first 20 seconds, your cheeks, chin and upper lip for the next 20 seconds, and then your neck for the final 20 seconds. Done.

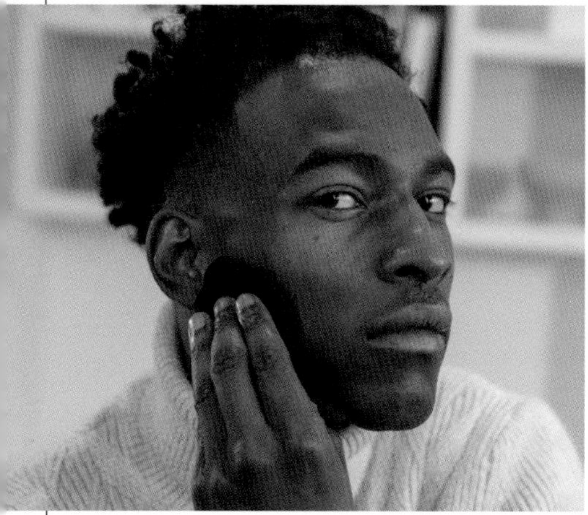

The deep cleanse: 3 minutes+

To go that bit deeper with your cleanse, try a double cleanse once or twice a week. As the name suggests, it involves not just one method of cleansing, but two. It's ideal if you regularly wear makeup. First, use a specific makeup remover or cleansing oil to gently lift off makeup and sebum build-up on the surface of your skin. For part two, follow up with a good, old-fashioned lathering cleanser using warm (not hot) water to get deeper into the pores and refresh your skin.

> **Tip**
>
> **You're going to use your hands to wash your face, right? If your hands are dirty, you're at risk of rubbing impurities directly into the skin on your face and defeating the object. Before you get to work on your face, thoroughly wash your hands first with a mild soap.**

Ditch the disposables

Time to get woke here. It's all too easy to reach for a face wipe to swipe your makeup off in seven seconds flat at the end of the day. What's the harm, right? Turns out, quite a lot. Single-use products such as wipes and cotton wool can take hundreds of years to break down, having a massive detrimental impact on our environment and ecosystems.

Before they were legally banned in October 2020, people in England were getting through 1.8 billion plastic-stemmed cotton buds each year with 10% being flushed down toilets and ending up in our waterways and oceans. While this ban is 'a drop in the ocean' on the giant war on plastic, it makes way for the takeover of reusable eco options. If you haven't already made the switch, it's worth considering....

Sustainable alternatives such as washable makeup remover pads and reusable cotton buds might not seem super-cheap from the outset, but their reuse potential means they're kinder to your pocket – and the environment – in the long run.

Reusable eco pads should last you around one to two years depending on how often you use them. We recommend having a stockpile of at least seven so you can use them and then stick them in your washing machine on rotation. Another option? Look for products that are biodegradable and compostable so you're still doing your bit. David Attenborough would be proud.

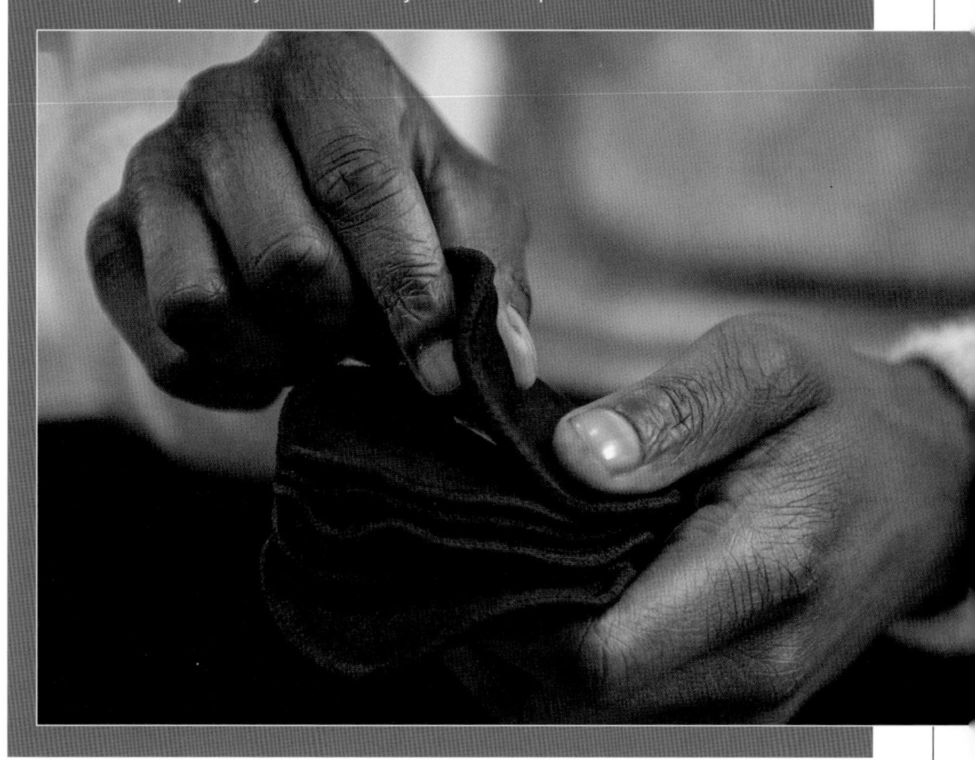

Makeup removal

What goes up, must come down. And in makeup terms, what goes on has got to come off. We get it. If you've rolled in at 1am from a big night out, the last thing you feel like doing is a full-blown skincare regime but, at the very least, always take your face off. Not only will it make you feel more human when your alarm starts buzzing at 7am, but it will keep your skin in check so you're not dealing with breakouts alongside your hangover.

Whether it's full-cover foundation or a light dash of concealer, sleeping in your makeup is a big no-no. Full stop. It can clog pores, and since sleep is a key time when your skin is doing its overnight repair work it needs to be able to breathe. If you want to keep your face super-fresh before you hit the sack, use a dedicated makeup remover and then follow it up with your usual cleanser.

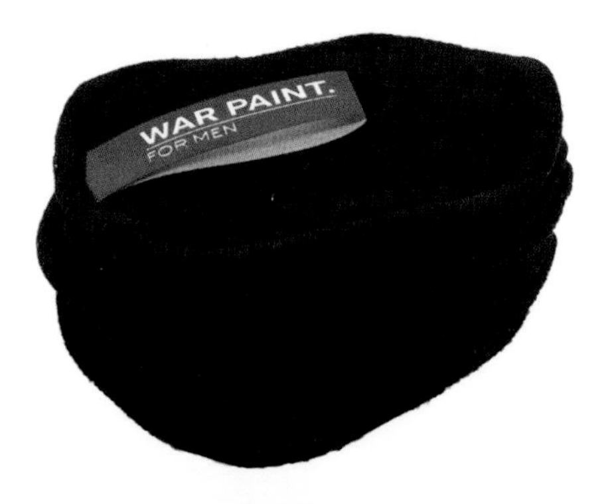

How to remove makeup

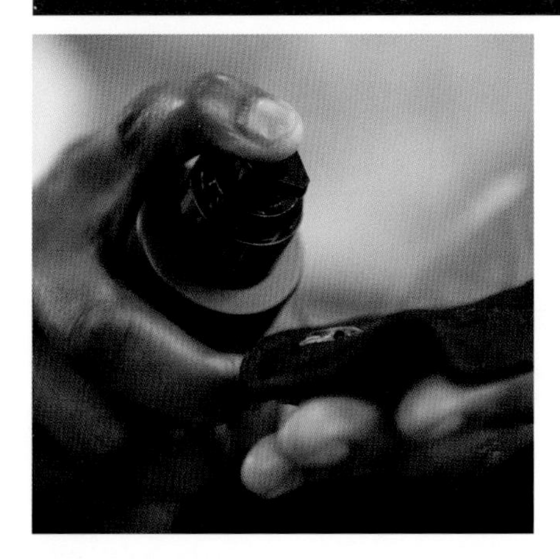

1 Pump a couple of drops of makeup remover on to a cotton pad.

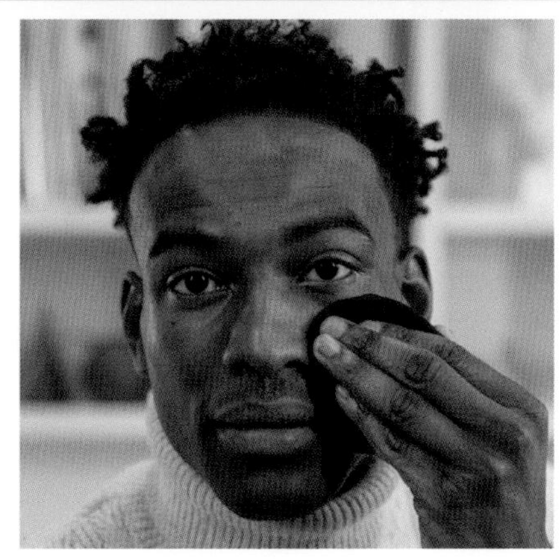

2 Gently wipe the pad across one side of your face to remove the makeup.

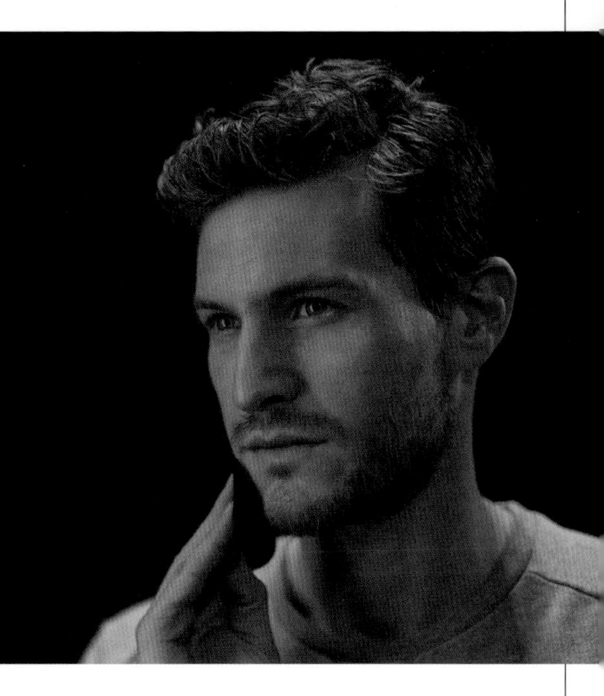

Tip

If your face is feeling 'squeaky clean' after cleansing, you might just be doing it wrong. Your skin shouldn't feel tight – that's a sign that your cleanser or facial wash is too harsh. If that's the case, put the bottle down and give your face a welcome breather.

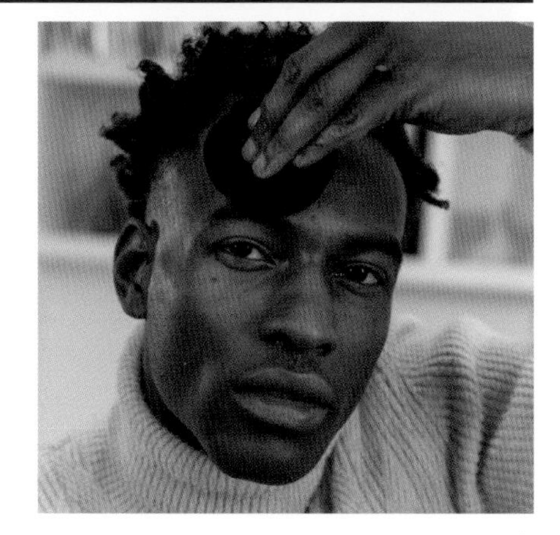

3 Repeat on the other side. Use a second pad if you're wearing heavier coverage or you feel like your face needs it.

Do and don't

✓ Do wash your face upwards and outwards to get a deeper cleanse (it's all to do with the way the follicles are orientated). The reverse is true when you're applying makeup, which you don't want to drive into your pores.

✗ Don't rub your face dry with a towel after cleansing. Instead, pat it gently. Being too aggressive with drying can lead to worsening of dryness.

Scan to watch the **'How to remove makeup'** step-by-step video

First published in February 2021

British Library Cataloguing in Publication Data
A catalogue record for this book is available from the British Library.

ISBN 978 1 78521 758 6

Library of Congress catalog card no. 2020943159

Published by Haynes Publishing,
Sparkford, Yeovil, Somerset BA22 7JJ, UK
Tel: 01963 440635
Int. tel: +44 1963 440635
Website: www.haynes.com

Haynes North America Inc.,
859 Lawrence Drive, Newbury Park,
California 91320, USA

Contributing author: Lisa Haynes
Content production lead: Ashley Fairfield
Additional images: Alia Haggag
Page design and layout: Richard Parsons
Photos: Alamy (page 16, 19, both); Getty (page 21);
Shutterstock (page 18, both)

Printed and bound in Malta

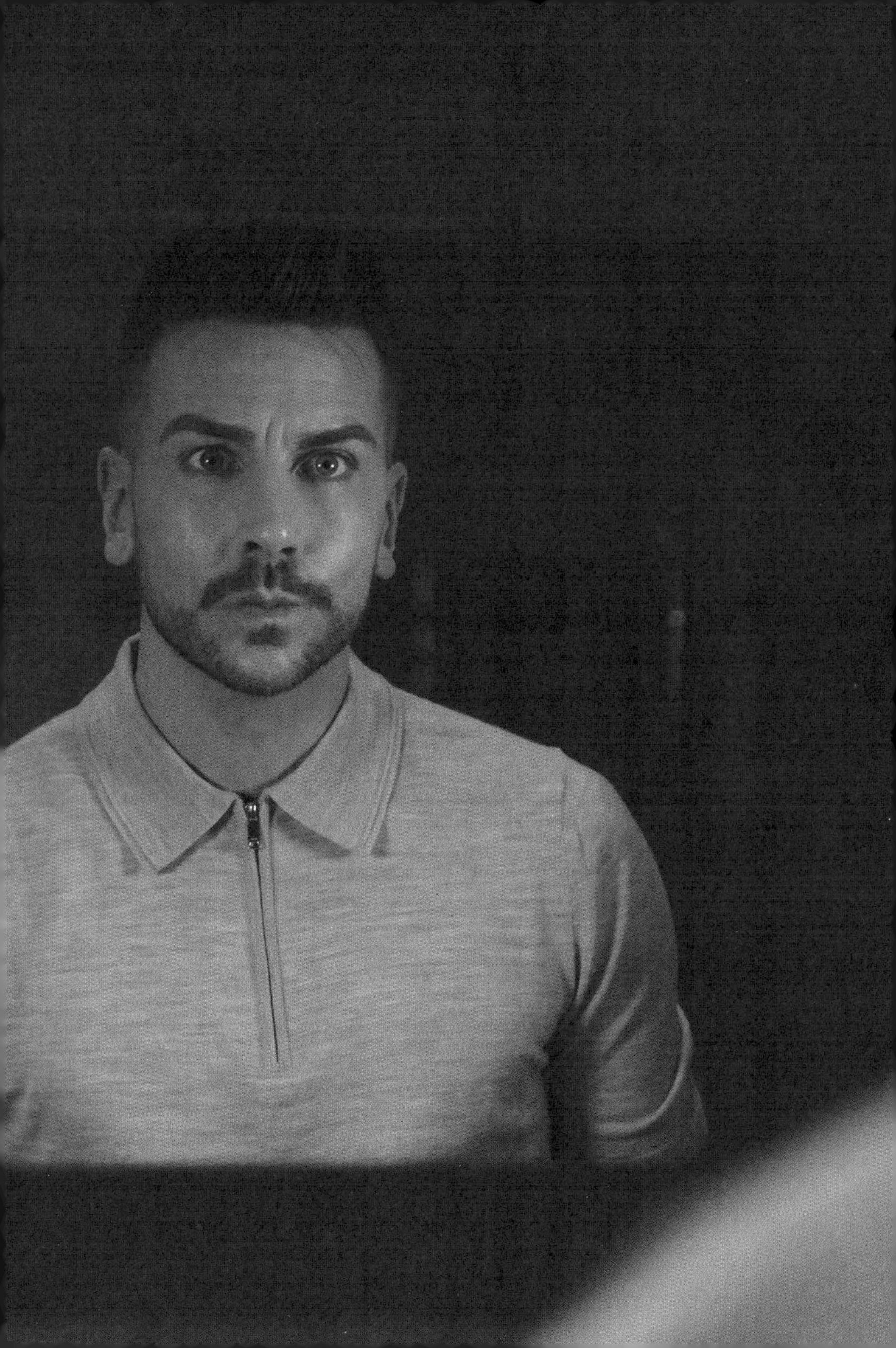